GLOBAL BIOETHICS – PERSPECTIVE FOR HUMAN SURVIVAL

Edited by **Brunetto Chiarelli**

Global Bioethics – Perspective for Human Survival
Edited by Brunetto Chiarelli

Published by InTech
Janeza Trdine 9, 51000 Rijeka, Croatia

Publishing Process Manager Sandra Bakic

Technical Editor Teodora Smiljanic

Cover Designer InTech Design Team

Additional hard copies can be obtained from orders@intechopen.com

Global Bioethics – Perspective for Human Survival, Edited by Brunetto Chiarelli
p. cm.
ISBN 978-953-307-537-2

For EU product safety concerns:
IN TECH d.o.o., Prolaz Marije Krucifikse Kozulić 3, 51000 Rijeka, Croatia,
info@intechopen.com or visit our website at intechopen.com.

Meet the editor

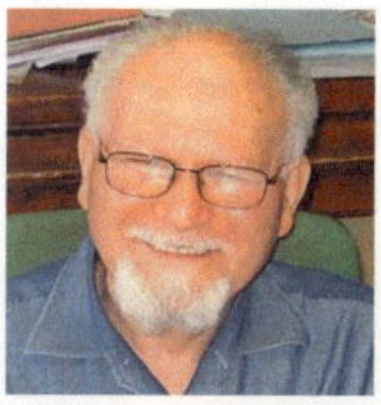

Dr. Brunetto Chiarelli received his degree in Natural Sciences and Biology from the University of Florence in 1958. In 1961., after two-year stay at the Institute of Genetics of Pavia, he was nominated as professor at the University of Turin where up to 1979. he taught Anthropology, Primatology and Human Ecology . In 1979. he moved to the chair of Anthropology in Florence. From 1970. to 1975. he was a Visiting Prof. at the University of Toronto, where he taught Human Evolution and, as expert of human cytogenetics and genetics, took part in the UNESCO project the "Human Adaptability", on the Eskimo population of Igloolik. He was past President of the European Anthropological Association, and present President of the European Association of Global Bioethics. He is the author of 400 scientific publications concerning problems of genetics, cytogenetics, Primate taxonomy and evolution, biology of present and past human population, and Bioethics. Chiarelli is currently editor in chief for following journals: " Human Evolution"; "International Journal of Anthropology" and for "Global Bioethics", a specific journal dealing with the human impact on Nature.

Contents

Preface

The collapse of Thomistic theology, followed by the development of scientism, positivism and mechanism of Nature, led to an unconditional faith in progress, with ideological crises that had also social and political consequences (Marxism).

Three new factors have since been added to the ideological change in the second half of last century: (1) The ecological impact of humankind on the environment; (2) The innovative impact of biology, which led to the decoding of genetic information annihilating our concept of individual and species as fundamental units ; and (3) The new biotechnological potentialities to produce food and energy which involve scientists and governors ethical responsibilities.

This stage of fundamental rethinking is however overshadowed by the threat of ecological disaster due to population increase, which undermine the very survival of Humankind. The biotechnological and biomedical ethical choices of human behavior depend from the interaction between human populations and the natural ambience.

Thus Global Bioethics, is concerned with defining clearly, the problems connected with how Humankind can best survive, at present and in future. It is an interdisciplinary Science that collects information from the traditional biological disciplines as Ecology, Ethology and Sociology, and places it in a philosophical framework with Man as its focal point.

Medical Ethics, must be considered as extension and modernization of traditional Medical Deontology.

A general theory for the evaluation of criteria for good and evil must in fact be first of all based on rational and naturalistic principles and must adopt the same criteria of Science.

Brunetto Chiarelli
University of Florence,
Italy

1

The Biological and Evolutionist Bases of Ethics

Brunetto Chiarelli
Laboratory of Anthropology and Ethnology,
University of Florence, Firenze
Italy

1. Introduction

A rational and naturalistic definition of ethical norms must stipulate the preservation of the DNA typical of the species and the maintenance of its intra specific variability. Indeed, this preservation is the basic principle of bioethics. The historically limited behaviour can be related to morality which can assume different norms in different historical contexts. Morality could therefore be governed by religion or normalized by discipline. Ethics, instead should be a purely biological and ecological discipline.

Religious ethics, medical ethics, political ethics, environmental ethics, business ethics, bioethics: a never-ending sequel of terms that began in 1892, when Felix Adler (1851-1933), questioning Christian and Jewish control of moral dogmas, established the Society for Ethical Culture in New York. Moreover, the terms moral philosophy and ethics are today often confused starting misunderstandings. So far, the development of ethical norms in western culture has been based on the distinction between theological ethics and humanistic ethics. Theological ethics follow Aristotle, according to whom everything has as an ultimate goal. According to this view, a contemplative life allows individuals to share divine life. The Stoics, following Aristotle, believed that living in accordance with Nature was the basis of moral philosophy, since they regarded Nature as a rational and perfect order being God himself.

Humanistic ethics base moral philosophy on human demands, primarily on survival. So it appoints moral philosophy to guarantee the survival of individuals or groups of individuals co-operating and living together in peace.

Ethical concepts are marked by duality because they can be either theological or humanistic. This duality peculiar to Western culture can now be overcome and integrated by a "global bioethics" with rational and naturalistic grounds, as required by the advances in scientific knowledge.

2. The historical, cognitive and cultural bases for "global bioethics"

On 11 July 1987 the Earth's total population reached 5 billion. Currently it is over 6 billion. In 1835 the figure of one billion was exceeded, thus in less than two centuries (or 8-10 generations) the human population has expanded more than six-fold. The current upsurge of the growth rate marking the turn of the millennium can be compared to the period of transition between the Paleolithic and the Neolithic (10.000-8.000 years ago), when the world's population rose from 5-10 million to over 100 million. The introduction of agriculture, breeding, fermentation and food conservation enabled Neolithic human kind to overcome the ecological crisis that had brought famine and despair to the hunters of the late Paleolithic.

Today it's a critical time when population growth and levels of raw material interact. Humanity will succeed in mastering this interaction only if a balance is found through intellectual faculties. Such a crisis can be overcome if the ethical problems concerning the applications of the biotechnology and genetic engineering, which call for quick and innovative decisions, are solved. Our knowledge has been revolutionized by the impact of scientific changes: firstly by nuclear fission, that changes the conceptual basis of matter; secondly, by the crisis of the concept of the individual, due to organ transplants; thirdly, by the development of molecular biology and biotechnology, of genomic information decoding, as well as that of "genetic engineering" undermining the very concept of species.

Will the development of "genetic engineering", that can yield energy and food, enable us to replace fossil fuels as a source of energy? Will bioengineering be able to produce cheap food to satisfy needs of a growing population? Will mankind be able to absorb the effect of these new technologies within a few years? What is going to be the impact of new technologies on the environment? What kind of world are our children going to inherit? As for governments, will they be able to manage such changes? How many lobbies will affect these choices? Will politicians be able to consider these issues in the short time left?

3. The self-consciousness of problems

The 1960s and 1970s were marked by a growing awareness of environmental issues and the critical relations between Humankind and Nature. This was the outcome of the critical remarks by scholars of various disciplines, including theologicians and philosophers, which gave rise to new cultural movements with a strong focus on environmental problems in the late 1970s. These remarks are summarized in the Stockholm Declaration on Human Environment (1972), that follows:

"We see around us growing evidence of man-made harm in many regions of the earth: dangerous levels of pollution in water, air, earth and living beings; major and undesirable disturbances to the ecological balance of the biosphere; destruction and depletion of irreplaceable resources; and gross deficiencies, harmful to the physical, mental and social health of man, in the man-made environment, particularly in the living and working environment".

Similarly, the solemn declaration of the Christian representatives gathering in Basel at the 1974 Council of European Episcopal Conferences reads: "Our *prosperity is mainly based on other peoples' poverty. We soil the world we live in with our selfishness and self-interest* ". The concept that the quality of life and the quality of the environment are closely connected, is confirmed by the final remarks of the UNEP Intergovernmental Conference on the Environment in Nairobi in 1982:

"During the last decade new perceptions appeared: the effort to manage the environment, the deep and complex interrelationship between the environment, development, populations and resources. Population growth, especially in urban areas, gave rise to social tensions. A global, region-wide approach stressing these relations is going to promote a sustainable development".

With his typical sharpness the Nobel Prize laureate, Carlo Rubbia (1984), said: "We are witnessing an experiment where the test tube is the Earth. Moreover, we can watch from inside, and nobody can guess what will happen". However, the development of genetic engineering also enables scientists to modify the human and other species genomes. In 1984, the Austin friar Arrano Rodrigo remarked: "For the first time in history a biological species is in a position to plan its own future by using its descendants as experiment tools". The well-known geneticist Francisco Ayala, (1985) wrote in support of this view: "Before the human race appeared no species could determine its evolution patterns; now humanity has the technical skills to do and maybe we can even direct genetic changes ". Which was echoed by Carlo Rubbia:

"*Now man claims he can change the genetic code. Let us consider we can plan, change and recognize the dualities of a person by his genetic code. We have not gone so far yet, for nature can still defend itself well. But man used to be tenacious in this field, so one day he will be able to modify the genetic code. This is an Aladin's lamp that we had better wonder whether it is worth opening" (1984).*

The words uttered by Francois Jacob in 1987, on the centenary of the Institute Pasteur, are also clear:

"*In the solar system nothing is more amazing than a cell turning into a man or a woman. It is a real wonder! Even science fiction becomes a stammering of imagination. A single cell, then a group of cells, then billions of cells. A universe where other cells are individualized so the human being starts speaking, reading, writing. I am bewitched by this. I would like to know the details... so far, genetic engineering has not been applied to man. We all agree that this must not be done. Biologists mistrusted first. The genetic values of man must be respected. There have been too little advances in scientific knowledge. If we want to make out what AIDS is, we must resort to genetic engineering. Each new discovery has a positive side and a negative one. When the Stone Age ends and the Iron Age begins the knife is discovered This is a useful tool, if you want to peel an apple, but it can be a deadly weapon as well. Nobody knows what science can achieve. Current forecasts are short-term, so they are uninteresting. Genetic engineering is a fantastic tool, but we must make a clear distinction between the atomic bomb, that is a bad use of science, and science itself*".

Therefore, it has become imperative to revise the idea of Nature exploited by Man and the common use of biotechnology. Humankind must manage environmental resources and his scientific heritage with a sense of responsibility. According to the aphorism by Galileo Galilei, "I *look for the light and for the benefit science can bring*". Scientific culture must revise its position by placing the training of scientists before that of technologists. Our relationship with nature is wrong, because the current establishment can neither raise conscious citizens nor upright statesmen. So we must find an ethic based on responsibility and solidarity as a requirement for human survival, as Hans Jonas (1990) Russel Van Potter (1971) maintain. The natural environment must be understood as a living system of which the human species is an integral part. Environmental awareness requires us not only to know the natural balance, but also to respect and recover it. This implies an attitude based on sharing and helpfulness replacing the exploitation peculiar to western culture. In this perspective, we must revise all our attitudes based on the exploitation of nature and the unlimited use of biotechnology. We must manage environmental resources and scientific heritage. Today's ethical problems are mainly noticed by biologists and natural scientists, but they affect all sciences and their solutions will be vital for all living species to survive.

4. The story of ethical concepts

In tracing the development of ethical concepts either a historical method or a naturalistic method can be followed. To date most scholars have followed the historical method. In order to understand how the concepts of good and evil, right and wrong developed and how they can be applied to our life, we can start from ancient Greece. Their systematisation started from things and was applied to Men; by following what we could call an experimental method a concept of good on a human scale was elaborated.

Ethics was in fact the third, highest branch of philosophy, alongside with logics and physics. According to this view men were also "things", and one's own happiness was the ultimate goal. Individuals had not to care about harming others, but only about their own pleasure: this was a hedonistic conception. The same process marked the development of concept regulating relations amongst men as well as those between men and things.

The original ethics involved human relationships, restrictions on personal liberty affecting the members of a social group (father and mother, son and daughter, husband and wife, etc.) and their own rights. The Mosaic law from the ten commandments summarizes these norms very well.

Western culture was deeply affected when the experimental bases of ethics were replaced by the metaphysical bases. This change started with Plato, according to whom the way to knowledge is a conversion to good. A leading role was played by the ascetical concept of the Neoplatonists, aiming at detaching themselves from this world and looking on a transcendental world. Ethics was thus affected by mysticism. These mystical trends were further developed by Christianity. In the Middle Ages, Christian ethics were unable to solve the contrast between Man and Nature, liberty and need. Christian moralists divided the world into two parts: good and evil, with the former being placed in some distant future (happiness, heaven, etc.). During the Reformation, free will was carefully considered, but contrasts between good and evil could be reduced only in part.

The ethics which then developed in the Western world affected relations between individuals and society. This is how law and its rules developed, included democracy, peculiar to Western culture. The philosophical theories of the early nineteenth century led to the utilitaristic and positivistic doctrines that spread into mid-central Europe. For example, Hegel's positivistic theory of history, (the rational and the real are identical) led to Marx's economic concept of ethics, (history has no moral sense and will has no conceptual value). But beyond the metaphysical barrier, the whole problem subsists. The natural world, as well as the concepts of good and evil, fair and unfair, right and wrong, obedience and disobedience, obligation and liberty must be clearly systematized. Current humanity, is constantly pervaded by such dilemmas, as it is thwarted by the responsibility of a continual choice and by the search for general rules to resort to.

The concept of ethics can also be analysed in a naturalistic and rational way, replacing a hedonistic/utilitaristic view of individual happiness as the only aim to pursue and a mystical vision of good as perfection to strive for. If the issue of ethics is founded on scientific bases this first leads to agnostic attitudes, then it excludes all branches of learning but scientific ones. Science is regarded as the only source of knowledge and the only way of considering reality. In this formulation the theological conceptions of ethics are meaningless. So we reach the bioevolutionist position peculiar to the schools of Lorenz and Wilson.

According to Lorenz, animal and human behaviours are "*functions of a system created and shaped by a historical and philogenetic* " (1978). According to Wilson, ethical values and physical characteristics may have developed and stabilized through natural selection, giving rise to a genetic evolution of moral predispositions. "*So in the human brain there are censors that affect our ethical premises unconsciously and deeply; these roots develop into the instinct of morality*" (Wilson, 1980). Yet in western culture there is no coding of ethics regulating the interaction between Man and the natural world. The relationship between Man and Nature, as Aldus Leopold asserts (1933), remains strictly economic. The Earth is regarded only as a property, and the rules regulating the relationship between Man and Nature only provide only rights and no duties. The extension of ethics to the natural environment is required by both evolution and the current environmental crisis. It is the third stage of a sequence where the first two have already exceeded.

5. The birth of bioethics and its naturalistic bases

Man, (i.e. the science produced by human evolution), now regards Nature as a liveable environment (ecology) and a process shaping him and all living organisms (comparative biology). "*A reflection of the mind on nature, where the mind is matter itself*" (Chiarelli 1994). Bioethics originates in this frame of ideas. The scholar who coined the term, Russel van Potter (1971), defines it as a science of balance between Man and Nature, a bridge for the future of mankind. Yet the actual inspirer was *A Sand County Almanac, with Other Essays on Conservation* by Aldo Leopold (1949). So it is by its very nature and its historical environment that bioethics must highlight the problems related to the best survival of Man, both as an individual and as a species, in the present as well as in the future. Bioethics expresses the concern within the relationship between Man and Nature and is an interdisciplinary science linking information from mainstream branches of biology, ecology and sociology. These are organized in a philosophical formulation focusing on *Homo sapiens* and forming an anthropological and naturalistic discipline *par excellence.*

Conversely,the approach of bioethics as medical ethics is different and incomplete, since it must develop as a broadening and updating of medical deontology. This discipline has to be regarded as that branch of global bioethics specifically dealing with the interaction between patient and doctor and between patient and society.

Bioethics, as a science, subtends a general theory for evaluating the principles of good and evil between co-specific beings and must thus be based on biological principles.

According to these assumptions, a definition of bioethics must primarily propose "*the preservation and propagation of the DNA peculiar to the species and the maintenance of its intraspecific variability*". This definition contains the basic principle of bioethics. In essence, all living things deserve respect and ethical regard, be they species, individuals or preliminary forms (spores, gametes, embryos) or products of cloning (cuttings).

Yet, these ethical reflections are dissimilar and have a different weight - depending on the various biological groups - since their ontogenetic cycles are different. This hierarchization of values is inherent to the evolution of life on Earth.

A biological entity marked out by an haploid structure of genes, as a bacterium, a gamete, a spore or a halophyte, is **the first hierarchical level** of bioethical note. Because it has only one filament of DNA it is subject to random changes (mutations) that inevitably lead to extinction. The fusion of the two haploid structures presupposes sexual reproduction and therefore meiosis, acting as a selector of random changes, most of which would have led the haploid entity to extinction.

The diploid entity is **the second hierarchical level** in the complexity of living forms marking life evolution on Earth, and the greater complexity of this stage must be regarded from a bioethical viewpoint. Yet ethical considerations are different depending on whether:

1. The diploid entity cannot survive on its own, as to embryos, or
2. its reproduction cycle is already completed, or
3. the diploid entity is formed by individuals whose life is unrelated to the transmission of specific DNA to descendants, as it happens in sterile castes of social insects, or

4. it is devoid of specific variability and its reproduction is asexual (cuttings, clones).

The biological entities in category I can seldom help in supporting specific DNA and its variability in future generations, because their life and development are conditioned by a variety of environmental factors which eliminate a large number of individuals. The same happens to the seeds of plants and to the fertilized eggs of sea animals, reptiles and birds that other animals use to prey upon, or the zygotes of mammals that do not succeed in settling in the uterine wall. This state of uncertainty perspective limits bioethical evaluation of these entities.

Category 2 entities are those that have completed their reproductive cycle, or whose reproduction is inhibited by different causes. They are biologically useless so their existence is meaningless from a strictly biological viewpoint.

Category 3 includes of sterile castes of social insects.

Category 4 - among vegetables and some animals one finds diploid entities (such as cuttings and clones) that cannot be called individuals because they are copies of parental DNA, i.e. genetically identical to the parental individual. These are devoid of individuality and do not allow the production of genetic variability through sexual reproduction.

Other species (e.g. higher animals) are of greater bioethical interest because they can be labelled "individuals", i.e. as biological entities distinguished by "uniqueness, indivisibility and unrepeatability" throughout their entire ontogenetic cycle. These individuals are the outcome of a fusion between gametes that were produced by the meiotic process of parental generation. The germinal line is potentially active in all individuals of the population. This is **the third hierarchical level** of life evolution on Earth. In such organisms, the preservation of the DNA peculiar to the species and its intraspecific variability are assured by precise rules of socialization. For stimuli lead to the: behaviour and socialization which preserve the DNA peculiar to the species and its intraspecific variability:

A. Parental care;
B. Reproductive behaviour;
C. Co-operation in searching for food;
D. Co-operation in defending the group

A and B are strictly dependent on the biology of the species, whilst C and D are related to the environment. As far as the latter group is concerned, we must insert a constant called k that is linked to the environmental conditions where the species or the population (or the individual) live.

These four factors (A, B, C and D), unrelated to one another, are the grounds of the bioethical rules of **the third hierarchical level.** These four stimuli can also be quantified as energy-giving consumption (calories) and as the amount of time invested to fulfill the bioethical imperative of the reproductive process or survival (time). This quantitative transformation enables us to formulate an equation. Its result, if related to the individual energy-giving consumption, shows the minimum and the maximum population of a given species that can survive in a certain area:

$$(A+B) + k\,(C+D) = \Delta$$

From a genetic viewpoint, Δ is identical to the concept of "Deme". This defines the minimum number of individuals in a panmixial local population that is needed to guarantee the genetic variability assuring survival for an endless amount of generations. This definition of the deme stresses that genetic variability is an essential requirement. Four conditions are required so that the frequency of genes in a population remains constant: 1) lack of selection;

2) panmixia; 3) lack of mutations; and 4) lack of differential migrations. So the minimum number of individuals required for a population to survive for several generations must take these four conditions into account. On the contrary, the maximum number of individuals of a population in a given area is related to its genetic and ontogenetic variability as well as to the means of support found in that territory. (So the population cannot be made up of individuals of one sex and of the same age).

Starting from this general formula (applying to all higher animals), we can easily deduce ones which can be applied to man and his cultural development, taking into account that they affect the environment, i.e. C and D. Thus, a new formula can be expressed by the following exponential function of human intellectual faculties (ei), which could be identified as a quantifiable event of human activity as the concept of space-time:

$$[(A + B) + k(C + D)]\, e^{i} = \sim H$$

The social and intellectual control of the environment in the natural system can be the qualitative leap leading to **the fourth hierarchical level** of ethical rules, those related to Man, his culture and his relationship with the environment. For these reasons, the minimum or maximum number forming the Deme can differ according to the environment in which human populations live and their historical background.

The interaction between man and the environment produced and constantly produces rules marking his behaviour throughout history (moral philosophy, customs, mores) and facilitate survival. Thus moral philosophy is that branch of bioethics dealing with the rules that assure the best survival of our species depending on various cultural and historical contexts. This survival is strictly connected to the aforementioned stimuli, i.e. the relationship between parents and children (A), the relationship between man and woman (B), co-operation in searching for food (C), co-operation in defending individuals and populations (D), all of which depend on the environment the individual or population inhabits. This interaction between the four ethical drives of socialization and behavioural rules shows an interesting link with the trine interpretation of brain suggested by Mc Lean (Chiarelli, 1995). While the behaviours and the stimuli of socialization indicated by A and B are governed or received by the reptilian brain, those indicated by C and D are mainly centred in the paleomammalian brain (limbus). Both these brain stratifications suffer the inhibitory, corrective and stimulative action of the neomammalian cortex. For instance, the knowledge acquired through imprinting can be controlled, as can those imposed by induced habits, usual behaviour, the trend to social and political conformism, behaviour and knowledge with their main seat in the reptilian brain. Analogical, critical and causal thinking is what distinguishes the neomammalian cortex, especially that of humans (tab. 1).

6. From bioethics to global bioethics

The moral and adaptation choices of the human social structure, including biotechnological and biomedical ones, are consistent with the above formulation and the interaction between human populations and their environment (traditions). Moreover, they must be unrelated to the influence of religious or political leaders, because these ideologies aim at power and disregard this balance; a balance which must be kept and improved for the survival of our species.

In fact, Nature may be oblivious to human survival because humans and other species are the result of evolution. However, man misuses his reproductive capacity and overexploits natural resources, risking to destroy both himself and other species.

Returning to demography, according to forecasts 2025 the Earth's population will, reach 10 billion. It will be catastrophic if this population is granted with Western-style living conditions (as is desirable); the human species will be unlikely to survive. As the world is tormented by economic, cultural and moral crises, becoming aware of this new phase is a pressing need. Bioethics aims at a balance between Man and Nature in order to assure human survival on Earth. A complex but useful challenge, that has to be contested and won within the third millennium. Even the birth and the abuse of the word "bioethics" stress that corrective interventions are urgently required. Van Potter and I established the journal "*Global Bioethics*" and I wrote the book *Bioetica Globale*, for this reason, to show a naturalist and anthropological distinction of bioethics from moral philosophy and medical deontology. In fact, the distinction between ethics and moral philosophy claims to discuss the problem of the choice between good and bad, i.e. what is allowed and what is forbidden. It aims at doing this rationally and by refusing the influence of humanistic culture. The issue of "ethical anthropocentrism" is linked to this new way of organizing daily life as well as to our future choices, so that the survival of our species is assured.

7. Notes and definitions

A rational and naturalistic definition of ethical norms must stipulate the preservation of the DNA typical of the species and the maintenance of its intraspecific variability. Indeed, the aim of preserving the DNA of the species and preserving its intraspecific variability is the basic principle of bioethics. A historically limited behaviour can be related to morality which can assume different norms in different historical contexts. Morality could therefore be governed by religious or normalised by discipline. Ethics instead is a pure biological and ecological discipline.

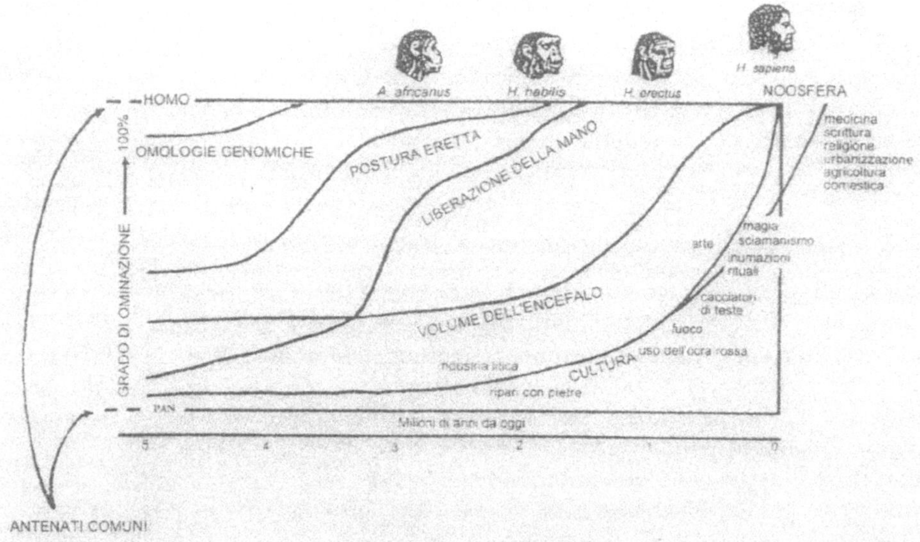

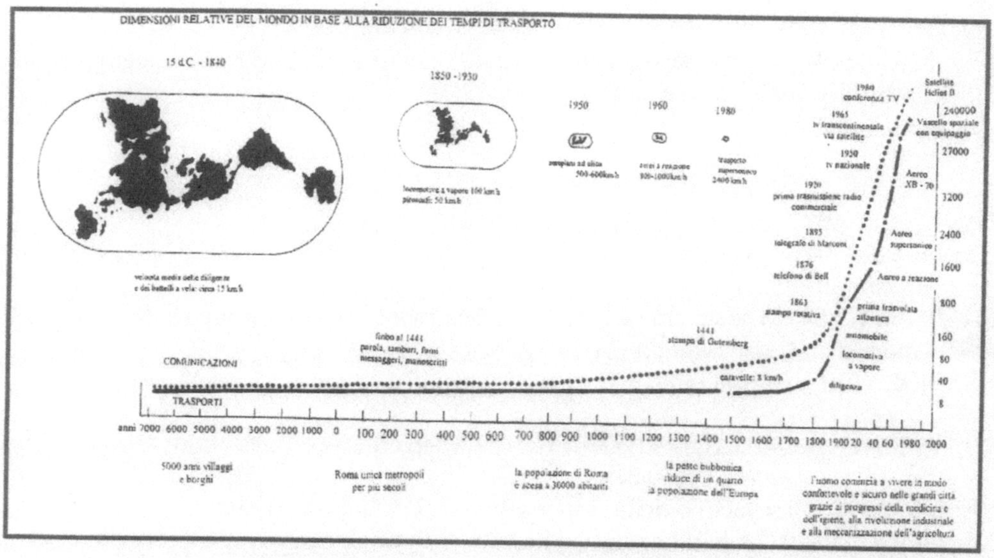

The definition of Bioethics: *"Preservation of the DNA typical of the species and maintenance of its intraspecific variability"*

Hierarchical order in the history of life and its ethical significance

1st level Haploid (n): microorganisms, gametes, spores, haplophytes

2nd level Diploid (2n): sexual reproduction (meiosis).

In this 2nd level peculiar ethical concerns must be reserved to the biological entities as:

a) cutting: they are identical copies of an original individual, as they do not have variabilities, they are produced asexually. It regards mainly cultivated plants and lower animals, now also artificial cloning in animals and possibly man (nucleo-transfer).

b) subsidiary class of social insects: they do not transmit the DNA of the species and they do not have reproductive potentialities

c) early stages of life as embryos and seeds: they have no certitude to reach the reproductive stage.

d) final stages as they have lost reproductive potential.

3rd level Diploid Biological Entities: with individuals which are unique, unrepeated, and indivisible.for the entire biological cycle.

4th level Vertebrate animals in which the maintenance of the DNA variability typical of the species and its intraspecific variability is assured by socialization defined by the interaction of internal and external factors (A: mother-offspring relation; B: sexual partner relation; C: cooperation in food research; D: cooperation in defence) and quantitative formula could be created to give the maximum and minimum number of individuals who could survive in a certain environment.

$$(A+B) + K(C+D) = \Delta$$

5th level Mankind in which the maintenance of the DNA typical of the species and to its intraspecific variability is assured also by the product of the brain activities (history, traditions etc). In this case Ethics can also become Moral Code as the four types of socialization input can be influenced by history.

Table 1.

8. References

Chiarelli, B., (1984), "Storia naturale del concetto di etica e sue implicazioni per gli equilibri naturali attuali", *in Federazione Medica 37:542-546.*

Chiarelli, B., (1984b), "Origine della socialità e della cultura umana", *Laterza, Bari*

Chiarelli, B., (1990), "Problemi di bioetica nella transizione fra il I e il III millennio", *Ed Il Sedicesimo, Firenze.*

Chiarelli, B., (1993), "Bioetica globale", *Pontecorboli Firenze.*

Chiarelli, B., (1994), "For a naturalistic definition of bioethics", *Social Biology and Human Affairs 59:8896.*

Chiarelli, B., (1995), "The carring capacity of the environment as it relates to reproductive morality", *Global Bioethics 8:149-157.*

Chiarelli, B., (1996), Le basi biologiche dell'etica e quelle sociostoriche della morale, *Biologia e Societa 1:19-20.*

Chiarelli, B., (1997), "A suggested distinction between ethics and morality", *European Journal of Genetics Society " 3:30-31.*

Jonas,I.H., (1990), "Il principio della responsabilità". *Ed. Einaudi, Torino*

Leopold, A.S., (1949), "A Sand County Almanac with other essays on conservation", *Oxford University Press*

Lorenz,K., (1978), "Natura e destino". *Ed. Mondadori, Milano*

Potter, V.R., (1970), "Bioethics: The Science of Survival", *Perspectives in Biology and Medicine 14:120153.*

Potter, V.R., (1971), "Bioethics: Bridge to the Future", *Prentice-Hall, Englewood*

Wilson, E.O. (1978), "On the human nature". *Harvard University Press, Cambridge, MASS*

2

How Ethics, Bioethical Thought, Laws and Restrictions are Imposed on Those Wishing to Donate Human Organs and Tissue

Eudes Quintino de Oliveira Júnior
Centro Universitário do Norte Paulista (UNORP)
Brazil

1. Introduction

The man is protected by the State from his conception. It is a modality of the American *welfare state*. During intra-uterine life the foetus is favoured with all the protection needed and if it is molested by abortive practices, those not considered legal, the agent of it will answer for the criminal action. If the mother, under the influence of the puerperal state, causes the child's death, it will be considered infanticide. The birth launches the child's reception in to society and the insertion of them into the protective measures of the infancy and youth legislation. On reaching the legal age, the citizen is covered by all the rights given by the constitutional laws and becomes a socioeconomic development collaborator of the collective, as well as developing strategies for their personal, familial and professional achievement. On finishing the labour period, they reach retirement and become a member of the Senior Person's Statute, which gives them a differentiated surplus of rights. In all the stages there is always exists the concern of the State in providing health conditions that are efficient.

The name transplant or transplantation is given to the surgical procedure which inserts into an organism which is denominated the host, a tissue or organ, collected from a donor. An Autotransplant, or Autoplastic transplant, is when the transfer of tissues is made from one place to another, in the same organism, as happens in the case of "bypass operations". Homotransplant or homologous transplant is when it happens between individuals of the same species. Xenotransplant is when the transfer of an animal organ or tissue to a human being occurs. Of course despite the progress of medical technoscience, Xenotransplants still need to accomplish a lot of tests to find a result that is considered satisfactory. More than that: if the project develops, many ethical problems will be eliminated because the human body will stop being the source of organs.

Man wants, at all costs, to prolong his life. It can even be a natural vocation to try to live more and, to do this, he tends to correct his imperfections to gain a richer existence, in regards to spiritual values, freedom, human dignity and social solidarity, and this is an eternal recreation. In order to live longer, besides therapeutic procedures, he also deems organs, tissues and other parts of his fellow man´s bodies, worthy. Medicine detects the sick organ, and, soon afterwards, through a reparative-destructor-substitutive intervention, it gets to manipulate a healthy organ, collected from another organism, correcting the one compromised in its functionality.

Biotechnology and biotechnoscience, with immeasurable advances, offer, in a short space of time, resources so that man can have not only his aspired longevity, but at the same time a better quality of life which gives a human person dignity, based on these self-established parameters he is able to reach his objectives. If the goal it is to reach a stage of harmonic life, very close to happiness, all efforts should be addressed towards this.

The human body, in this way, becomes a repository of tissues and organs, but it is clear the state will interfere in the disposition of the person's will regarding the donation of their organs in vita or post mortem. The availability of the body has its limits and can only happen when, for therapeutic and humanitarian ends, the necessity of the case must be clear. Even though it requires the sacrifice of one body in favour of another, the progress of medical techniques make a replacement possible with considerable margins of success.

Such an objective, by itself, causes an increase in the need for the supply of organs for transplant, because the number of people on waiting lists is far superior to the organ supply and it causes the rise of the black market trade of human organs. Despite the World Health Organization (WHO) rejecting the parallel trade, which observes the rule written in the Universal Declaration of Human Rights regarding the sense that the human body and its parts are *extra commercium* goods, without any trading profile; it is well-known that there is a growth of groups centred on illicit activity. Therefore the permission for the accomplishment of a transplant should obey rigorous criteria, with tireless legal control.

The donor, that transcends their own human nature, accomplishes the noblest humanitarian action, just like a pelican that makes free their blood to feed their nestlings. In this principal, the person, in a certain way, not only exposes themself to risks, but renounces the integrity of their organism to help another, in both cases with the state approval. Between physical integrity and human dignity, the Law supports the latter, because the altruistic disposition of the body, perfectly justifies the necessary state.

The impression is that when it comes to mentioning the subject of organ transplants the individual feels an attack on their body, identity and dignity. But, in reality, with the evolution of medicine and the progressive pace of the patient in taking a decision in regards to the new therapeutic perspectives, the action of transplant is integrated into the citizen's life, presenting itself as a solution for many chronic diseases until then incurable. The simple exercise of study or research does not warrant the sacrifice of a healthy body and of course when all conditions are analysed, the removal of an organ is only recommended to replace another that is compromised, taking into account the beneficence principal, consolidated in the *malum non facere.*

In the same way that, in therapeutic treatments the patient's autonomy prevails, the availability of the body, the parts and organs are, with equal reason, governed by the individual. Once the body belongs to them, they could, when they are lucid and conscious, direct it towards any purpose they judge convenient, regarding a therapy of no major importance. But, in reality, they do not have exclusive possession of their body. If they are above legal age, capable of taking decisions, they will freely be able to dispose of their body for therapeutic ends or for transplant in a spouse or consanguineous relatives until the fourth degree. If they intend to benefit another person, they should obtain judicial authorization, to avoid the parallel commercialization of human structures.

Like this, once again, the prevalence of the state interest occurs, to the detriment of the citizen's individual will. It is not referring to a prohibitive rule, but to the discipline of the procedure. The individual´s intention to donate organs to a determined person post mortem will not have any sway, because the will that prevails is the State´s, which will regulate and indicate the patient to be benefitted. It is also not a "nationalization of corpses", but a way to ensure the correct distribution of organs and human tissue to the registered people who await a transplant in order to have a chance at a worthy life. The principal of equality before the law or the equality among people is put into practise, whilst also taking into account the gravity and urgency of the disease.

The human body is an organ repository that can accomplish the substitution with considerable margin of success, providing man, on being done, a better quality of life. The thinking being can be its own wolf, but the corpse presents itself as an offering of organs to whom so needs. The donation, in its essence, is the act that transcends human generosity and it can happen, ironically, that the organ that is transplanted becomes an enemy of the donor. Without forgetting that modern technology makes the connection of devices to organs and human tissues possible, as in, for instance, artificial hearts, pace-makers, etc., which are attached to the human body by electronic circuits.

All of these considerations will be approached throughout this present study that had, as its basis, an analysis of the Brazilian legislation and the specific regulations applied to organ donations in vita and post mortem, as well as the criminal procedures that can be perpetrated in the process of receiving and distributing organs. Brazilian legislation respects and gives prestige to organ donation and creates safety mechanisms to correctly reach the purposed objectives.

But, if on one side there is the opening to favour the donation of organs, tissues and human body parts, transforming the donor in life into the licensee, there are also imposed limitations to this. In the same way, if in life they intended to create public or private documents anticipating their will in donating their organs, in post mortem the manifestation of this, will have no validity, because for the documents to be legitimate they need the authority of the relatives and spouses.

The reiterated transformations of medicine, which are constantly evolving, oblige the creation of more laws to attend countless solicitations that continually arise in the field of transplants. New strategies in capturing donators, always of a voluntary nature, also favour the understanding of society. The country is seeing a significant growth in the accomplishment of transplants, with highly significant results, proven by data officials.

2. The ethics

Ethics is the human being's moral line. Many thinkers and philosophers have unveiled into society their definitions of ethics, however, each time the concept has been presented in different apparel. This is due to the changeable nature and dynamic character of ethics, which evolves according to social transformations. But the central idea embedded in the word's etymology keeps its essence, emphasizing it as a lineal thought, with its eyes always facing forward, tracing a straight line, without any swinging movement, in the search for new harmonic spaces to be inhabited by man. Through its Greek origins, "Ethikós" symbolized the way of being, the character, the morals, and the good habits of an individual. So much so, that, in its original application, it was demanded of those who were engaged in public activity and representatives of the *res public* ("public issue" or "public matter") carers.

According to Oliveira Júnior, "Ethics still isn't concluded, it is a thought in constant evolution, which in the course of time, keeps improving. Ethics is not the result of codified

conducts, it does not revoke, nor is it repelled, even partly. It is the result of man's own evolutionary thought, which, in his essence, searches for happiness and perfection."
Therefore, the human sensor is able to know how to detect precisely when a certain kind of behavior, conduct or procedure fits into the established molds accepted by the community. The individual´s evaluation receives the homologation of the collective in relation to previous ethical approval. By rule, whatever is good, necessary and convenient for man, gets the *placet* from the community and starts to integrate itself into the way of life, without any restriction.
Ethics carries two propellers: one of them, collective, where the thought becomes one and widespread, this is a result of reiterated common-law practices that consolidate from generation to generation. Man himself transfers the concepts he received by adopting it and passing it forward. Another propeller is the individual, where the intimacy sphere establishes its own evaluation criteria and acceptability, which, can even be contrary to the common thought, but reveals the person´s status of independence and autonomy.
Autonomy is consistent in life's regent faculty. It comprehends the familiar, social, professional and spiritual existence however it does not cease to be an ethical achievement and in addition a revelation of free-will that reigns among beings endowed with intelligence. The will is a preponderant factor in which man affirms himself as a thinking and independent being. Oneness is the form in which man presents himself before a social group and acquires the quality of a human being and in so doing becomes known, for his virtues, attributes and imperfections; it is a vital characteristic in the valorization of human beings. At the same time that it is an indivisible and irreplaceable unit, the human being carries the universal seed of his genetic patrimony, which will ensure the continuity of humanity.
The creative Law of Humanity's Ethical Progress projected by the Spanish philosopher Marina marks itself in an intelligent way and without contestation:
"Any society, culture or religion, when it is liberated from the five obstacles - extreme poverty, ignorance, fear, dogmatism and hate of one´s neighbour - heads for a common ethical pattern, that is characterized by the affirmation of individual rights, the fight against unjustified discrimination, the people´s participation in political power, the initiation of rational dialogue, the legal and political guarantee of assistance".
Descartes´s famous philosophical saying, "*cogito, ergo sum*", translates in an unequivocal way the fusion between the being and the knowledge, it puts value on the human intelligence, the space where human beings cogitate and decide. But this premise can be considered true as an introduction to philosophical thought, however judicially it cannot prevail by reason of the principal of equality before the law that grants equal treatment to all people. It cannot in any way conclude a "contrariu *sensu*" that the person that does not think, the mentally deficient, for instance, does not exist. Regarding the removal of organs, tissues and other human body parts for transplant and treatment ends, the law no. 9434/1997 presents a correct and coherent assertion in which it establishes, as obligatory, in the 3rd article:
"The *post mortem* removal of tissues, organs or human body parts destined for transplant or treatment should be preceded by the diagnosis of encephalic death, verified and registered by two doctors who were not participants of the removal and transplant teams, by the use of clinical and technological criteria defined for resolution by the Federal Council of Medicine."
The human body, in this way, is nothing more than a clinical instrument, a perfect articulation of the biochemical and organic system, regulated by the decisions of the brain

that becomes the actions commander of the nervous centre. A true Dom Quixote like shield-bearer. It brings to mind the sincere and realistic narration made by emperor Adriano a Marco, in Yourcenar´s work: "This morning, for the first time, the idea occurred to me that my body, this faithful companion, this safe friend and more my acquaintance than my own soul, is nothing but a sly monster that will end up devouring his/her own owner".

Szaniawski observation is also pertinent, comments on and concludes the Spanish's lesson by Antonio Borrel-Maciá, in the sense that "the right to dispose of one´s own body would be subordinate to the norms that determine the use of the things. "Livestock" should be used and the power of disposal is governed in agreement with its nature and purpose. Identically, the use of the human body should be according to its nature and purpose, conserving the individual, in relation to this fact, his/her free will and his/her moral responsibility. The intervention of the legislator would only have as an objective to limit or denouce the practice of material or juridical actions that they constituted a social danger".

Within this view, man is the curator of his own autonomy. Although not entirely, because the concept of liberty on the whole is ambiguously independent. For us to say that liberty reigns in its philosophical concept is an excessively utopian idea as it needs to establish limits among people in order to promote social harmony. What remains is the individual 's internal liberty which due to being located in the intimate exclusive sphere cannot be invaded, however, it appears outwardly, passing through the filter of social acceptance and it can be contradicted.

3. Bioethic thought

The person's autonomy of will appears as a necessary consequence of *principium individuationis* and receives bioethic assent that institutes it as one of the basic principles. The New Science had its roots hurled into the debate in the year of 1947, in the Nuremberg Trials, in reason of the reflections related to the barbarities perpetrated during the world wars involving research using human beings, without any criterion and authorization. In the following year the Universal Declaration of Human Rights and the Nuremberg Code were edited, creating documents which generated a new age for the rights of the individual and collective, with a more dignified and human dimension regarding the person. The expression "Bioethics" was introduced for the first time by the oncologist Van Rensslaer Potter, in the book *"Bioethics. Bridge to the Future"*, in 1970 and it presents itself as a multidisciplinary universe with the purpose of discussing various aspects of human life through plural reflections, in order to generate transforming interventions, more appropriate and convenient for mankind to reach his objectives, as in the concepts established by Aristotle when he idealized the "supreme good".

The conscious will, that it is the result of a coordinated operation by the brain, forms an ideomotriz action that is nothing more than the accomplishment of conducts in favour of the person, as well as exerting the function of social life. It could even affirm that it awakens the consciousness of the human being's purpose. Its mind and body are interlinked and both are promoters, when in interaction, of the quality of healthy and harmonic life. The space of the humans' coexistence implants general rules and has the power to discipline the individual's behavior. This is the law exercising its primordial function of regulation.

But the individual will cannot be put upon by the established rules of society. It should be, before everything, respected so that it always prevails in the interests dictated by the community. "Everything in nature, made explicit by Kant, acts according to laws. Only a rational being has the capacity to act according to the representation of the laws, that is, according to principals, or: only he has a will. For to derive the actions of the laws, the reason is necessary, the will is nothing else but the practical reason."

The "*principium individuationis*", is the one that proclaims the predominance of the individual's will which is not absolute and nor can it be, in a society that is composed by numerous individuals. Each one owes respect to the other and freedom will only be reached when the same social objective is reached by all. In that respect the German philosopher Adorno, founder of the School of Frankfurt, proclaimed, with a lot of authority, the following:

"Sometimes the individual opposes himself against society as an autonomous being, although private, still capable of rationally pursuing his own interests. In and beyond this phase, the question of freedom is a genuine one for knowing if society allows the individual to be as free as they promise him/her to be; and, with that, the question is to know if he/she really is so".

To incorporate the political animal, as Rousseau defines it, man needs to receive the necessary tutelage against aggression and interference in his/her intimacy, protecting him against any abuse; in particular the state power should actively participate in the choosing of the rules that will regulate their conduct in the social environment to form the general will and to be detainer of the necessary financial conditions for the satisfaction of the fundamental demands of material life, for the fulfilment of a worthy life and to respect, above all, his/her freedom.

The constitutional proposal of the democratic State of Rights was instituted In this same principal with the purpose of "... to assure the exercise of the social and individual rights, the freedom, the safety, the well-being, the development, the equality and the justice as supreme values of a fraternal society, pluralist and without prejudices... "(Preamble of the Constitution of the Federal Republic of Brazil)

The continual progress of medical researchers, the medical-surgical instrumentalisation, the formation of highly specialized teams, the search for new alternatives for decreasing, stabilizing and even curing various diseases that afflict humanity have put in prominence the human body, transforming it into an inexhaustible source of replacement tissues and organs. The human body acts as both the donator and the receiver, through the surgical act denominated as the transplant, which inserts into the living host organism a donated organ or tissue. It is in the new medicine that on one side emerges the destructor of a sick organ and on the other, triumphant in its functionality, it reemerges as the one that substitutes and mends.

The philosopher Aristotle dedicated a great part of his work to biology and added to the body, the illustration of the human soul figure, which becomes the shape of the body, and strives to affirm that the soul cannot exist independently of the matter. "The body which the soul gives form to, is not, however, any matter; it is the form in relation to the tissues and organs, without which, it would not be this "organized body that has the life in all its potency", the one in which the soul, that is the culmination of a hierarchy of forms, comes to give life and takes it".

4. The autonomy of the will

The corporeity comes to express the singular reality of mankind. It is him who is the owner of a patrimony called the human body, detainer of its acts, administrator of this inexhaustible latifundium, that comes overlaid with a special tutelage that gives to it personality and turns it into a subject of rights and obligations. At the same time that it is an individualized patrimony, it suffers interference regarding its entire utilization. In a more convenient expression and attending to a more recent concept of "man´s-body", we can say that "...for body (the word body) we understand it as that dimension of Mankind in whose base it institutes itself into the structure of empiric entity. In this sense, it is something that can be observed and something that can be the aim of experience, whether on its structure or on its behavior. However, it is not about a local collocation, an extrinsic, but the radical and original, in which it has defined its origins and constitution, its maintenance, its decline and its end".

The new Code of the Brazilian Medical Ethics, introduced by the Resolution of the Federal Council of Medicine no. 1931, of September 17, 2009 taking in to account the world thought that governs the subject established a truthful and active communication channel between the doctor and the patient. The inquiry, which is constantly reiterated, tries to discover to where the autonomy of the patient's will goes to. It is known that the doctor is endowed with a specialized knowledge in a certain area and their word is of vital importance for the effective, low cost solution of the presented disease in a minimal time. It can, sometimes, not coincide with the patient's opinion who opts for a certain procedure, due to the existent liberty in the "Pacient Self-Determination Act". This decision partnership that is formed regarding the most appropriate treatment is nothing more than the conjugation of the alternatives of actions presented by the doctor and the free and autonomous choice of the patient. If, by fortune, it is announced that there is only one possibility for treatment, there is nothing to say about the exercise of the right of the autonomy of will. It is a peremptory decision, it does not accept another choice accepting of course the patient´s refusal of the suggested treatment.

This way, in the circle of his autonomy, man, in theory, is the lord of his own body. This is a reckless affirmation because he cannot make use of or dispose of it in some specific situations. The Universal Declaration of Human Rights proclaims in itself that the human body and its parts are *extra commercium* goods, which is reiterated in the Brazilian Constituition and the common legislation.

The availability of the body, analyzed through the viewpoint of bioethics, is possible, but only if you follow the basis and principles of both autonomy and beneficence, there is an existing agreement from the donor, the purpose is therapeutic or humanitarian, and reverts itself into a significant benefit with a minimum risk. There is a severe evaluation between the assets that are in play and the proportionality of what is more beneficial and this will dictate the right conduct of behavior.

Every capable person is gifted with ample conditions for managing his/her actions in civil matters. The individual can do whatever is allowed and no one can be obliged to perform what the law does not command, according to the constitutional (article 5º, II, CF). What occurs is that the public power (the ruler or government) imposes restrictions on the people whilst also granting relative freedom.

The Brazilian Federal Constitution, after ensuring that health is everyone's right and the State´s obligation to maintain it, thoroughly establishes in regard to human organs removal the following, in article 199, paragraph 4:

"Law provides the conditions and requirements for the removal of human organs, tissues and substances for transplants, research and treatment, as well as the collection, processing and transfusion of blood and its derivatives; whilst prohibiting any kind of commercialization".

The man as an end and value in himself, a centre and point of convergence for all of the actions, endowed with a volitional and intellectual capacity, detainer of his own supremacy, exerts in his condition as moral subject, with a personal decisive autonomy, looking for all of the means for the development of his inalienable dignity. Therefore the Federal Constitution, when it establishes the Federal Republic objectives does not make any distinction regarding the human being, considering the equality within him and prohibiting prejudice against origin, race, gender, colour, age and any other discrimination forms. (Article 3rd, parenthesis IV of the Federal Constitution).

The text reflects the constitutional legislator´s concern in specifying in only one paragraph various conducts involving the transplant of human organs. In the first plan it appears that organ removal will only be allowed when the purpose is for the realization of a transplant, research or treatment, if they are within the patterns proposed by the common law, which will establish all the conditions and requirements. In the second, it makes it clear that the collection and processing of blood and its derivatives will be managed by the loose law. In the third, the prohibitive rule is inserted that will be reiterated at a later point in the legislation in a sense that any kind of commercialization of the material collected is prohibited.

The progress and evolution of society, its habits, the incessant development of research in to human beings, the beginning to the end of life, the choice of the child's sex, human cloning, genic therapies, methods of aided human reproduction, substitutive maternity, eugenics, euthanasia, dysthanasia, orthotanasia, the choice of the time to be born and to die, genetic engineering, gender reassignment surgery in cases of trans-sexuality, the use of DNA recombinant technology, the use of the embryonic stem-cells, transplant of organs and human tissues, biotechnology and many other scientific progresses that are not mentioned here, have opened an immense sphere of medical actuation, mainly in the research and laboratory area. New technologies that seem unattainable are offered to the big medical centres and they are made available for use in human beings. The perplexity crosses the boundaries of curiosity and it causes the creation of a new field where it merges together medical ethics, bioethics and human volition, all in search for the definition, direction and solutions for their conflicts. It brings to mind Pitigrilli, in their unforgettable book "O Homem que inventou o amor" (The Man that invented love)", when it prophesied that as much as medicine as much the right have the need for mountains of victims to progress a few meters.

The whole summation of the technological resources exercise direct influence in man's evolution, turning him, from generation to generation, into a more refined specimen containing the databases of his species. This deposit of information reveals the environment in which his ancestors lived and it provides a guide to survival which is more suited to the rational of human nature. "What is special about DNA, affirms Dawkins, proclaimed in 2005 as the most influential British intellectual by Prospect magazine, teacher at Oxford University, England, and author of fundamental works on 'evolutionary biology,´ is the fact that it survives not in its own matter, but in the form of an indefinite series of copies. As occasional mistakes of copy happen, new variants can still survive even better than their predecessors, and like this the database with the information that codify recipes for survival gets better through the course of time. These improvements will show in the form of better bodies and other resources and solutions for the preservation and propagation of the codified information. In essence, the preservation and propagation of the DNA information will usually mean the survival and the reproduction of the bodies that contain it.

5. The legal restrictions

The Brazilian Civil Code (Law n. 10.406, of 10/01/2002), in its turn, in the chapter that deals with personality rights, describes in the sole paragraph of its article 13, the following rule:
Art. 13. "Except for medical demand, the act of the disposal of our own body is prohibited, when it results in permanently diminishing it´s physical integrity, or contradicts good customs".
Sole Paragraph. "The action described in this article will be admitted for transplant purposes, in the form established by special law".
The rule is the prohibition *in vita* of the disposal of the body that belongs to you, according to what can be deduced from the legal text, in the cases that cause any damage to the physical integrity or resist the rules of good customs. It is the prohibitive commandment like rule of the exercise of disposal of our own body. It puts an end to any questioning in regards to the absolute property of the body, unless it is due to medical exigency, which, in addition, must be previously delineated by the State. If, from one side, there is the individualized legal tutelage of the citizen, from the other, there are restrictions imposed by reason of the moral and ethical objectives deriving from the legislation.
The legal permissive inserted in the paragraph points to the realization of the transplant, in the pattern established by special law. The understanding of the written law is that our bodies are unavailable to us, being accepted, as an exception, the intervention by means of a transplant. The State would present itself, in this circumstance, as a co-owner of the individual body.
The organ and tissue donations in Brazil are regulated by the Law, number 9.434/1997. In the *intervivos*, where any capable person can consent to, or in the situation where they are unable to, his or her legal representative can, as long as they are double organs (kidneys, for example), or renewable parts of the human body, for therapeutic purposes or for transplants for a spouse, consanguineous relatives until the fourth-degree, or any other person, depending in this case on judicial authorization; being exempt from this only is the case of a bone marrow transplant. The donation must in every account be free in reason of the orders within article 199 § 4th of the Federal Constitution and the Law 9.434/97, in its 1st article.
The legal norm appears to be that the *inter vivos* donation is allowed, since the purpose is the accomplishment of transplants or therapeutic ends, as long it is about double organs or renewable parts of the body, involving a capable person, or his/her legal representative for the due authorization and that the beneficiary is the spouse, or consanguineous relatives until the fourth degree. If it is for someone that is not from the specified family, there is a need to obtain judicial authorization, as the consent of the capable person or his/her legal representative no longer has any value. But if the person who will donate is judiciously unable, even after his/her immunological compatibility has been verified in the cases of bone marrow transplant, despite the authorization of the parents or the one legally responsible, it must follow that judicial authorization should come as a *plus* guarantor of the action. And, if in the case that one of the genitors is declared absent, the other will request judicial consent for the other genitor in their place.

The availability of the own body in its altruistic purpose seeks, on one side, to protect and to limit risks to the donor and, on the other, to avoid eventual commercialization of organs. But the law, which may have been edited with a certain urgency, may have forgotten to contemplate the donation of human organs and tissues in the cases of adoptions.

Regarding the free disposal of the own body, *post mortem*, it is established in article 14 of the Civil Code:

"It is valid that, with a scientific or altruistic objective, the body can be freely disposed, in the whole or partly, after death.

Sole paragraph: "The act of disposal can be freely revoked at any time."

The donation *post mortem*, in its turn, will be executed with the spouse's authorization or a capable relative, in the familial line straight or collateral until the second degree, and the law demands that the responsible medical team declare the patient's encephalic death, in reason of the ceasing of the cells responsible for the central nervous system. It remains, however, that the heartbeat, indispensable for the removal of organs or tissues continues. The Law n. 9.434/97 defined the concept of death, adjusting it to the encephalic failure and not to the biological life, governed by the heartbeat. The ancient romantic ones used to put the hand on the chest to watch the beats of the heart. Today, rationalism rules it. Without encephalic activity, there is no life. The pulsing of the heart is irrelevant therefore, if life has already abandoned the body. In this there is nothing further to discuss about the practice of euthanasia if encephalic failure has already been declared and the doctor has turned off the life support device that maintained the patient's biological activity.

Brazil regulated that the beginning of human life starts with the conception *in uterus*, meaning therefore, when it regards *in vitro* fertilization, with the manipulation of the masculine and feminine gametes and the consequent freezing of the embryos, there is no life but a group of reproducing cells. From the moment that the transfer to the uterus happens, the *spes vitae* begins. Death happens in reason of the bankruptcy of the encephalic activity, permitting from this point the announcement of the human organs and tissues for extraction.

Law demands that the act has to be representative of human solidarity, always encased in gratuitousness. Otherwise, it would be open to the possibility of accomplishing the trade of human organs and tissues, attracting so called investors through the trivialization of the human being. Sometimes, it can be seen in newspaper announcements that a person puts up for sale, alleging financial need, one of his/her kidneys, leaving their address for the negotiation. A legal project was discussed, through legislative process, to make it possible for the convicted to serve as an organ donor and in exchange he/she would receive commutation of his/her sentence. These are situations which conflict with the ethical principle that surrounds the human being in his/her dignity by depreciating the human race. Man continues being his own wolf, in Thomas Hobbes's expression.

The rigorous legislative demand has its foundation in the control of the medical procedure that, based on the principle of justice, it provides everyone with the right to receive human organs or tissues, independently of his/her financial situation. Otherwise, only the favoured ones would have access to the regenerative procedure. Even so, with such rigidity, the system has been manipulated and organs are diverted to patients that are not on the waiting lists, or, if enrolled, they do not occupy a primary place. It is a true criminal task that, to reach its aims, it counts on the active participation of some health professionals who should care about an efficient way for the reception process and insertion of organs, should strictly obey, the donor list for the ones that have been in the queue for a long time awaiting the procedure and, with preference, those in a more precarious health situation.

The Medical Ethics Code *(Resolution of Federal Council of Medicine n. 1931, of September 17, 2009)*, in its article 44, demands that the doctor responsible for a procedure is obliged to enlighten the donor, as the receiver, or, if it is the case, their legal representatives, of the current risks of the exams and surgical interventions in the realization of the organ transplant. Such determination marries with the bioethics principle of the patient's autonomy of will.

It is interesting to observe that the law that regulates transplants has determined a donation presumption, known as the "silent consent", which is, that every person would originally be a donor, unless he/she expressly manifested on his/her Identity card or on the National Driving License, with the expression: "not an organs and tissues donor". In so being, the donation is an act of human solidarity and is spontaneous, it cannot be coerced.

In order to eliminate the obligatory nature of the previous law, in the Law n. 10.211/2011, the following was made explicit:

Art. 4th "the removal of tissues, organs and parts of the deceased person's body for transplant or other therapeutic purpose, will depend on the spouse's authorization or the relative´s, over the legal age of maturity, obeying the successive, straight or collateral line, until the second degree; as well as the provision of a document signed by two witnesses present at the time as to the verification of the death."

This way, if the person in life, left registered document in the sense that he/she intends to donate his/her organs *post mortem*, it is possible that a revision of the decision on the part of the relatives, could be made to annul it entirely. This demonstrates that the autonomy of the person's will, suffers severe limitation in putting himself/herself as an eventual donor. The Brazilian Civil Code, in its article 1857, allows the realization of the testator's will, that, in possession of a sound mind, establishes the disposal of the totality of his/her goods or part of them and even regarding non-patrimonial will, in the case, for instance, of child's recognition or of stable union. In this, his/her will is respected and executed. This is not valid, however, regarding post *mortem* donation of organs.

The encephalic death will be declared after the termination of neurological exams done by two doctors that are not participants in the reception teams or transplant, being one of them a neurologist or neurosurgeon. It comes regulated by the Resolution n. 1.480 / 1007, of Federal Council of Medicine. After this, the notification will be made to the Notification, Reception and Distribution of Organs Headquarters, that it will be responsible for the indication of the receiver's name, properly registered.

All health establishments are forced to notify the reception headquarters of an encephalic death occurrence. If the authorization has been checked and the establishment is not accredited to do the human organ or tissue removal, it should allow the patient's removal or, if this is impossible, to franchise the access to a transplant medical-surgical team and those responsible for the removal of organs.

If, in life, the patient manifests that he/she had the intention of being an organ donor, the relatives feel more comfortable in deciding to sign the medical term of consent. Otherwise, it will always be more difficult and it will demand the formation of a family committee to make decisions regarding the donation. As it is known, in practice, it is not a good moment for making such an important decision, because, at the same time as there is the announcement of encephalic failure, the body registers vital signs and there is the impression that they are being asked to rush the death, through the practice of euthanasia.

There are a considerable number of patients without a chance of recovery that are not sought by the specialized medical teams in the announcement of encephalic death. According to data from the Brazilian Medical Association Magazine, about 60% of the population agrees with organ donation, however intensive care professionals and emergency services notify just one out of eight potential donors.
The rational of law rests exactly in this crucial point. Through the principles of proportionality or of reasonability, a death is decreed when a body no longer responds to excessive therapeutic appeals and it gives prestige to the other patient who has a real possibility of recovery and will be able to live their life to the full. For this, there has got to be a need for efficient work regarding the decreeing of encephalic death, not meaning in so doing, the extirpation or elimination of human life, pure and simple. But with the necessary professionalism and above all, with the awareness that a death is already announced by a knowledgeable medical professional, it is to give resurgence to the other life, by reason of the consented donation.
The relatives are extremely connected by the family bond and are not prepared to reflect on the donation of organs, for even comprehensible reasons. When the encephalic death is announced, the relative knows that the body is being moved by driven biological propulsion and there is always the hope of revitalization.
The organ donation campaign in Brazil is still timid in its transmission of advertisements, as to the providences to be taken by the relatives. It is right that the most important providence is the dialogue between them for making a concerted decision and in agreement with the will of each one, before the event of death. However the public appeal for the donation to a certain person is forbidden. In relation to the appeal for funds to finance the transplant or graft, the National Management organization should make understandable campaigns and explanations regarding the donation of organs.
The president of the Brazilian Association of Transplant of organs, Bem-Hur Ferraz Neto, in his end of year message to the class, with a clear sensation of unrestrained hope, regarding the reached results manifested himself as such: "In the year of 2010, ABTO started a new challenge, the one of knowing the results of transplants accomplished in the Country, in which it refers to the rates of patient and graft survival. The only way of obtaining success in this was to stimulate our associates to make this challenge their own, which we did through a vigorous campaign and e-mails. We finished 2010 with a quite favourable allegiance with the associates and transplant teams, but we still cannot say that we know all the data, exception being the pancreas transplants and pancreas-kidney, because these teams communicated 100% of their results. Therefore, these teams deserve our congratulations and the recognition of a commitment to the society".
Berlinguer e Garrafa mention some forms in which people are persuaded into donating organs: "In a Congress that had the theme Ethics, justice and the trade of transplants, the Transplantation Society described, in 1990, five possible ways of obtaining living people's organs: a) relatives' donation; b) donations from people emotionally linked to the receiver; c) donations with altruistic ends; d) paid donations; e) aggressive trade."
The Tribunal of the Justice of Rio Grande do Sul had an interesting initiative to receive through a link in its website the personal information of donor candidates which could later be printed in the format of a certificate. Of course the document, by itself, is not covered by validity; however it is enough to represent the person's will and intention before the relatives.

The project Transplant Living, being worldwide, has the appropriate recognition. Known by the acronym U.N.O.S. (United Network for Organ Sharing) it is a non-profit organization and maintains the National Corporation of Harvest and Transplant in direct cooperation with the Health Resources and Services from the United States Department of Health and Human Services.

The Public Health System in Brazil is the biggest promoter of transplants: it finances about 95% of it, besides also financing immune suppressor medicines. According to the Brazilian Medical Association, Brazil is "the second in the world for renal transplants losing out only to the United States. When that number of transplants is presented in relation to part of the GDP, Brazil is the one with the highest performance in the world".

The auto-transplant was also contemplated in the legislation and it would only be possible to accomplish if the individual offers his/her authorization in a consent document, or if the person is judicially unable or is not in a favourable health condition, the consent will be given by one of the parents or someone legally responsible.

On the other hand, the consent of the receiver or of his/her legal representative if he/she is judicially unable or does not possess the conditions for manifesting his/her own will, enrolled already on the waiting list, after taking into account the exceptional nature of the measure and of the risks of the procedure, will be offered in a free and illustrious way.

When the corpse is not identified or claimed by the public authorities, in the period of thirty days, the Law n. 8501/1992 rules on it, assigning it to medical schools, for teaching means and scientific research.

6. Illicit penalty

The Law n. 9.434 / 1997, maintaining the penal rule of the *lex specialis derrogat a lex generali*, also establishes a charge of criminal premeditated conduct, when the agent has full knowledge of the illicit character of the fact, and other administrative ones.

It is like article 14 expresses:

To "remove tissues, organs or parts of a person's body or corpse, in disagreement with the dispositions of this Law:

Penalty - reclusion, from two to six years, and a fine of 100 to 360 a day."

It is noticed, in the reading of the text, that the core of the penal type is sustained by the verb to remove, that, in its origin expresses a movement back, to arrange to remove something from a place, to remove, to take, to suppress, and to separate. In the case *sub studio* it means the transfer that is done of a certain organ from a person to other. Therefore the legislator was careful in differentiating the removal *inter vivos* and *post mortem*. The first of them demands the living person's manifestation or of his/her legal representative, while the second, the relatives' consent. As it is a crime that can be practiced only by those that have the legitimate right to remove organs, tissues and parts of the human body; the members of the transplant team who perform the procedure will be held criminally responsible.

It is an absolute certainty that the *ratio legis* seeks to prohibit any removal of tissues, organs or parts of a person or corpse, without obeying the criteria established in law. In this, the *contrario sensu*, filled out the legal conditions, that, the action is lawful, because it is supported by the law. The Code of Medical Ethics, already referred to, in its article 45, instead of using the verb "remover", it opted for the verb "retirar", both, however, have the same meaning.

Article 15 of the law that disposes of the removal of organs, tissues and parts of the human body for transplant ends and treatment, prescribes it like this:
To "buy or to sell tissues, organs or parts of the human body:
Penalty - seclusion, from three to eight years, and a fine of 200 to 360 a day.
Sole paragraph. It incurs the same penalty on those who promote, intermediate, facilitate or gain any advantage from the transaction."
The act of buying or selling referred to by the legislator comprehends the illicit practice of trade acts, having as a reference the *res*, the *pretius* and the *consensus*, in the acquisition and sale of tissues, organs or parts of the human body. The illicitness of the action consists of contradicting the prohibition of considering the human body as a trade object. Contractual freedom is an instrument recognized by the law that allows a party to circulate private wealth and grants authorization to one of the parties to transfer the goods of his/her property to another person. But the goods that he/she intends to trade should be viable and judicially possible for the business to receive the seal of the State. When it refers to organs, tissues and parts of the human body, they are considered *extra commercium* goods, removed from any commercial initiatives. Regarding organ trafficking in Brazil it is recommended to read the book Kidney for Kidney, by the publisher, Record, in which the researcher Júlio Laudemir presents an interesting report on foreign and Brazilian people involved in the black market and illegal trade of human organs.
The penal responsibility does not only centre on the people who accomplish the purchase and sale, it can even be the health professionals, but it expands and it reaches to other people that direct or indirectly, in any way, promoted, intermediated, facilitated or gained any advantage from the transaction. The intended benefit is not just exclusively financial, but any other one that results in earnings or benefit .
Article 16 describes it as the following:
To "accomplish a transplant or graft using tissues, organs or parts of the human body whilst having the knowledge that it was obtained in disagreement with the dispositions of this Law:
Penalty - seclusion, from one to six years, and a fine, from 150 to 300 a day."
The type of charge in question is aimed at the professionals that accomplish a transplant or graft and that have the knowledge in advance that the organs, tissues or parts were obtained illicitly. Despite the consciousness of the illicit conduct, they premeditatedly accomplish the medical action regardless. Interesting to notice that the special law did not predict this guilty conduct, in the areas of incompetence, imprudence or negligence, and because of this the transplant can only be accomplished in the field of legality by being a procedure that should be followed strictly, phase by phase, with conscious adhesion to the accredited medical team.
Article 17 emphasizes:
To "collect, to transport, to keep or to distribute parts of the human body in the knowledge that it had been obtained in disagreement with the devices of this Law:
Penalty - seclusion, of six months to two years, and a fine, from 100 to 250 a day."
The *voluntas legis* strays away from those that accomplish the transplant act and it invades the performance sphere of those who are in charge of collecting, transporting, keeping or distributing parts of the human body. It is an illicit act practiced through multiple conducts seeking to reach the professionals that, although they do not accomplish the fact, are subject to a more serious penalty, develop other activities that will favour the illegal transplant. The

accomplishment of a conduct already characterizes the crime. He/she is an offender, the agent that has a full knowledge that the parts of the human body that are being collected, transported, kept or distributed, were obtained in an illicit way, without obeying the established criteria of law.
Article 18 proclaims:
To "accomplish a transplant or graft in disagreement with the determination in the art. 10 of this Law and its sole paragraph:
Penalty - detention, from six months to two years."
The law intends to protect the patient having in its sight the principle of the receiver's autonomy of will, giving him all of the necessary information regarding the exceptional nature and the risks of the procedure. After being properly enlightened about it, he/she will sign the consent that authorizes the conduct.
The protection is extended in the cases in which the receiver is judicially unable or when his/her condition of health restrains or prevents his/her freedom to express the valid manifestation. The law demands that the consent can be supplied by one of the parents or one legally responsible.
Article 19, finally, emphasizes:
To "fail in recomposing the corpse and returning him/her to their rightful aspect, for burial or to fail to give or to delay his/her delivery to the relatives or interested parties:
Penalty - detention, from six months to two years"
The crime therefore highlights the need for tutelage in the respect of the dead and their relatives. Despite the fact that it is a corpse, without human life, it preserves all the affection of the family and friends. The *ratio legis* of a crime occurs when the corpse is submitted to any procedure for organ extraction or even forensics and the responsible professional does not return it in the rightful physical aspect, that is, with his/her normal human appearance, so that it is buried and remembered like this by the relatives and friends. In the same way the professional is punished who does not return the corpse, without justified reason, of course, or delays its delivery to the relatives. In both actions, it is configured that the illicit act has as its passive subject, the relatives of the dead.

7. Conclusions

The scientific evolution means that man is getting closer to life longevity. Man is not searching for immortality like the character Conde Fosca, who overcame death in the book "Todos os homens sao mortais", by Simone Beauvoir.
Man is aware of his finiteness and intends to prolong his existence, making use of therapeutic resources and even of the several modalities of transplants of organs, tissues and human body parts.
Ethics and bioethics monitors this and will establish the limits of reasonability. Ethics, being responsible for the correct conduct, which is socially adjusted, searches for a harmonious approval of the procedure. Bioethics, for its turn, will analyse if its reparative conducts through the transplants are necessary and convenient for man. It would be a balance of the cost and benefit, always giving prestige to the margin of safety and warranty for man, in the limits of the *primum non nocer*e.
The judicial positioning, finally, will regulate and execute the ethical and bioethical thoughts, consecrating them in a pattern of laws. It is known, from when Montesquieu

wrote "O Espirito das Leis", that the law exercises a restrictive function and, at the same time, a cogent one, in order to assist its social purposes.

The autonomy of the person's will suffers limitations in the legislation regarding the transplant. If, in the civil area, the person has the freedom to affirm public or private documents regarding donation of their goods or even recognition of an illegitimate child, with total legitimacy and acceptability, the same action of will does not produce any effect regarding organ donation.

There is clear state intervention in preventing excessive donations in vita and post mortem, in agreement with legal order. Besides the legal requirements pointed out for the transplant realisation, those who are health professionals or their auxiliaries and even others that in a conscious way, defraud its rules will be subject to a criminal process, with the application of the restrictive penalties that incur the loss to the right of freedom. Such restrictions appear as inevitable and have the purpose of avoiding the illegal practice organ and human tissue trade.

But, even like this, as is shown in the presented graphs, transplants in Brazil are demonstrating an expressive growth, with the unquestionable tendency of extensively overcoming the numbers reached up until now.

The fact that the community is now understanding the restrictions imposed on their autonomy of will with regards to what they can and cannot do, as well as the specialization of more receiving and organ distribution teams and the authorization granted to the other centres to practice these procedures, are all indicative factors of the approval and good results reached by the transplant teams in Brazil.

8. References

Revista Brasileira de Hematologia e Hemoterapia, vol. 31 - Suplemento 1 - May, 2009, page 157/164)

Marina, José Antonio, O quebra-cabeça da sexualidade. Rio de Janeiro, 2008

Yourcenar, Marguerite. Memórias de Adriano. Rio de Janeiro, 2005

Theodor, Adorno. Dialética negativa. Rio de Janeiro, 2009

Dicionário dos filósofos. Denis Huisman - Publication Director. São Paulo: Martins Fontes, 2001, page 69

Dicionário de Bioética. Editorial Perpétuo Socorro. Editora Santuário. Under the direction of Salvino Leone, Salvatore Privitera and Jorge Teixeira da Cunha for the Portuguese language edition, August 2001, page 207

Dawkins, Richard. O maior espetáculo da terra: as evidências da evolução. São Paulo, 2009

Rev. Assoc. Med. Bras. vol.49 no.1 São Paulo Jan./Mar. 2003

Canotilho, José Joaquim Gomes. Direito constitucional e teoria da Constituição. - 7ª edição. Portugal: Livraria Almedina, 2003, p. 268

Revista Registro Brasileiro de Transplante, year XVI, no. 4, jan/dec 2010

Berlinguer, Giovanni; Garrafa, Volnei. O mercado humano. Translation Isabel Regina Augusto, Brasília: Publisher - Universidade de Brasília, 2.ed., 2001, p. 124

Revista da Associação Médica, vol. 49, no. I, São Paulo, jan/mar.2003

3

Help and Coercion from a Care Ethics Perspective

Guy A.M. Widdershoven[1] and Tineke A. Abma[2]
[1]*VU Medical Center EMGO+ institute/Depart of Medical Humanities,*
[2]*VU Medical Center EMGO+ institute/Depart of Medical Humanities,*
Amsterdam,
The Netherlands

1. Introduction

At present, there appears to be a tendency to attribute (shared) responsibility to (healthcare) professionals, such as medical doctors, parole officers, mental health care workers and child services employees, in questions of safety. At times they may be asked to alert the police or other authorities in order to protect the safety of their patient/client or his environment. This raises the question of what you would do, as a professional, when you suspect your client becomes involved in criminal activities or neglects or abuses his housemates.

In such cases, professionals are often hesitant to inform the authorities. They feel they ought to respect the autonomy of their client and should not invade his privacy. This reflects our common belief that help and coercion are contradictory and conflicting values. Autonomy is one of the core values in our Western culture and equated with independence and freedom of choice (Widdershoven, 2000; Verkerk, 2001). Within the context of health care self-determination is also considered an uncontested right. The idea of the self as free and independent mirrors itself in the shift from the patient as a passive recipient of care to the patient as a 'consumer' or 'critical customer' (Emanuel & Emanuel, 1992; Thorne & Paterson, 1998; Guadagnoli & Ward, 1998).

Yet, the question remains whether not interfering or not steering the client is in fact the optimum way to respect the client's autonomy. To what extent can one speak of autonomy when we close our eyes and allow someone to get involved into criminal behavior? From the viewpoint of the professional should one not attempt to change the client's mind, stimulating him to engage in different activities, deliberately preventing him from such behavior? Indeed, should one perhaps even consider employing persuasive or coercive tactics, even if this includes restrictions in the freedom of the client?

In this article, we propose and recommend a view of autonomy based on the ethics of care (Tronto, 1993; McKenzie & Stoljar, 2000; Verkerk, 2001a). Herein autonomy does not equal self-determination and self-ownership without the interference of others, but is defined as the ability to direct and shape one's own life based on and in relationships with others. From such a perspective, actions of third parties may actually be necessary to enhance autonomy. Autonomy is thus not understood in opposition to relations of dependence and connection. A relational conceptualization of autonomy in which vulnerability and dependency on others are considered to be part of life and constitutive of autonomy helps to find legitimate ways to intervene in the lives of clients.

This does not mean, however, that every manner of intervention is justified. The issue is not whether or not an intervention is indicated (legal perspective), but how this intervention can be shaped so that the people concerned feel empowered and supported by it (ethical perspective). We illustrate this relational view of autonomy based on the ethics of care with a case description from a primary care organization for people with a physical or intellectual disability in the Netherlands.

2. Case MEE

MEE is a Dutch primary care organization for people with a physical or intellectual disability. Part of their client population consists of young adults (under 30 years) with mild intellectual disabilities who live independently and who sometimes have so-called 'double' difficulties as they also suffer from behavioral problems or personality disorders. This group can be highly impressionable and is often found to be involved in a variety of criminal behaviors, such as growing hemp plants, illegally claiming cars and dealing drugs. Especially those with double difficulties frequently end up in the justice system. This may entail involvement in a wide range of sometimes serious or violent criminal activities. Part of this population has been the topic of case discussions in local safety houses where representatives of municipal, judiciary, care, and welfare organizations have gathered to devise strategies on how to deal with these adolescents and young adults. To facilitate discussion, the participating organizations are expected to share all relevant information about this group of youngsters including to the department of justice, when illegal acts are involved.

Counselors at MEE are habitually confronted with facts that point to the (suspected) involvement of their clients in criminal activities. They may see a weapon in their rooms, smell marijuana plants in the attic, find stolen goods, etc. At times clients may even talk to their counselors about their illegal behavior or there could be other clues that something is going on, for instance when there suddenly is a lot of money or expensive equipment in the house, while the client does not have any financial resources.

The police expect MEE counselors to report these situations or file a case when appropriate. However, the counselors hardly ever do this. This can be explained by a number of factors. For example, they may feel it is not be the job of the professional to report someone. After all one is there to provide care not to act as a policeman. The protocol for social workers also states that such action is not indicated. In this protocol, the importance of the client and particularly the respect for his privacy is emphasized rather than the importance of society or general interest that is served by reporting the crime. The counselors also have their own opinions on the behavior of their clients: they may not always feel it is that bad. This differs amongst counselors (i.e. where one feels more strongly about the presence of marijuana plants than another). In addition, some counselors may feel it is not (always) their business. They consider the presence of, for example, stolen goods in the clients' house not to be part of the professional contact/interaction they have with the client. They are, in their opinion, no detectives and feel it is not their job to find out if something is wrong or acting illegal. In other words, only when the client himself reports involvement in illegal activities is there a possible role for the counselor. However, even in that case, most counselors do not feel they need to report it to the justice system. On occasion they may confront the client themselves, at other times they confer with colleagues or they take no action at all as they feel they do not have to or cannot do anything. Sometimes counselors may also be afraid to speak up about what they see. As a result, oftentimes counselors do not do much about the signs and suspicions that their clients are involved in criminal behavior.

3. Two approaches to autonomy

In ethics, autonomy is often identified with self-ownership and self-determination. Somebody is autonomous when he or she can decide for himself what happens. Following John Stuart Mill (1859), autonomy as self-ownership describes the freedom of the individual to shape his own life unhindered by others. His renowned principle of freedom/liberty holds that an individual is sovereign in directing his own life, as long as his actions do not hurt others. Notable authors in the field of health care ethics have emphasized that respect for autonomy means that the health care professional should avoid meddling in the decision making of the patient or client (Beauchamp & Childress, 1994). When the client is attracted to criminal behavior, one should not intervene unless his safety or that of others is at stake/in jeopardy.

Non-intervention is stressed in this view of autonomy. The individual is to rule about his own life without interference from others. This is considered negative freedom/liberty. The concept of positive freedom/liberty can be distinguished from that of negative freedom/liberty (Berlin, 1969). It deals with an increase in freedom/liberty in the actions or choices of people. Positive freedom/liberty focuses on a person's ability to be the source of his own decisions and to lead his life in accordance with his own value-commitments, goals, and plans. In the positive notion of freedom/liberty not only the question whether people can make their own decisions, but the content of these choices is also taken into account. From the standpoint of autonomy as positive freedom/liberty one does not have to respect every choice. A choice that is in accordance with the life-plan of the individual has greater importance than a choice based on a random impulse (Dworkin, 1988). The ethical value of the continuation of one's life path and personal history can also be found in the work of Ricoeur (1992). People become incredible, untrustworthy and irresponsible when they step outside their life history, and cannot keep up the promises they made to others. So when someone engrosses himself in criminal activities this does not signify/exemplify autonomy, because the choice is not an expression of what the person truly values in his or her life (unless the person made a clear and informed choice to engage in illegal activity). Yet, even such a deliberate choice becomes questionable if it, for instance, implies that the client can no longer be responsible for his family. Think of a patient who is addicted to alcohol or drugs and can no longer care for his son.

Care ethicists adhere to the notion of autonomy as positive freedom/liberty (Verkerk, 2003). They stress that autonomy is not the same as independence. Autonomy can only be developed in relationships with others, so in situations/states of dependence. Hence care ethicists speak of relational autonomy (MacKenzie & Stoljar, 2000; Verkerk, 2001a). From a deliberative perspective people require support to gain insight into what is important in their lives and how to arrange their lives accordingly (Oeseburg & Abma, 2007). It is not always simple to choose friends. Sometimes one needs to be warned not to be tempted into an (seemingly) alluring situation. When one lets people in vulnerable circumstances choose their own company, this does not prove of respect for their autonomy but of neglect. By helping them guard themselves against 'wrong friends' their autonomy is actually reinforced. Help and support will not be limited to this. The client's criminal activities afforded him a particular role and might even have given him a certain status level. Besides money and material goods, criminal activities in itself are valued in certain communities. Therefore, finding alternative ways to a respectful life are crucial in the cessation and prevention of illegal activities. From a positive view on freedom/liberty, care professionals should help their clients (or refer them to others who can help the client) to discover better ways to participate in society and live a meaningful life. This implies an active search for pursuits or pastimes that fit his personal wishes and abilities. In addition to developing a daytime program, care professionals should also assist their clients in attaining a different social network. Lastly, clear and achievable agreements should be made based on joint discussion (such as no longer socializing with certain people or frequenting certain meeting places). Informing the healthy network of the client may be helpful/effective in this. Family members and acquaintances can remind the client of the arrangements. Care professionals can also check regularly whether or not clients have kept their promises, and if not, why not, and try to adjust/improve the situation accordingly. In this way care professionals help to empower their clients.

According to Agich (1993), individuals are never fully formed but they are part of a dynamic process of development, in interaction with their environment. Only for a person without an identity does freedom/liberty mean absolute independence. Dependency need not impair anyone's freedom/liberty as long as that person can develop and mature. The same holds true for the mutual influence that care professionals and clients have on each other. As stated by Agich, it is more important to help clients to live with their vulnerabilities and to accept their limitations (for isn't this what it means to be human?) than it is to offer them freedom of choice (Agich, 1993). This means that it is more important to guard people against the temptations of criminal activity, then to let them do whatever they want.

4. Inducement and coercion

From the perspective of care ethics, respect for autonomy constitutes more than not interfering in the decisions of the client (Verkerk, 2001b). Sometimes it is necessary to influence the behavior of the client, especially to be able to add to their autonomy as self-development (as opposed to autonomy as self-determination). One can execute inducement and persuasion in an attempt to change the client's mind or even employ coercive measures to prevent negative consequences. We speak of inducement when a client still has the freedom to make a choice (e.g. if you do not stop growing marijuana plants, then I will have to report it to the police). In the case of coercion the client has no choice (e.g. I will get the police involved now).

Care is a process of negotiation and corresponding perspectives. In this context, Moody (1992) coined the term 'negotiated consent.' According to him, care does not merely consist of offering information and waiting for consent, but reaching a joint understanding through negotiation. Care professionals cannot simply sum up the risks and wait for whatever the client decides to do. This is unfair, especially when clients are missing the cognitive or emotional intelligence to value and weight various alternatives and to oversee the consequences. By being involved with client the professional should (attempt to) encourage the client to handle risks in a responsible way. This means that they should enter negotiations with the client by actively offering and discussing their options.

Moody (1992) points out a number of ways in which health care professionals can intervene during the process of negotiation. He discerns four types of intervention. The first is *representation of interest*. The professional works as an advocate for the interests of the client and tries to defend these. For this their interests must be understood. And if necessary the care situation should be adjusted, for example when a client does not want to be helped by a certain professional, but only by another. The second form of intervention is *stimulation*. Here, the objective is to encourage the client to look at himself differently. For example, start to see again that one is a father with responsibilities for a family instead of just being a alcoholic and patient. The third intervention is *persuasion*. The professional tries to persuade the client to comply/be cooperative by offering convincing reasons. These must be tailored to the client's circumstances. The fourth and final intervention is *deciding for the other*. In this situation the client no longer plays an active role. According to Moody, though, even in this case is there communication and negotiation, for example with the family, or between professionals.

What does the approach of Moody mean for the care professionals at MEE? First of all, they need not accept every form of conduct from their clients. They can try to convince their clients to show more responsible behavior. This could consist of modifying the situation they are in (for example by giving someone a daytime activity or removing them from a certain environment) or through the strategy of stimulation. A client is then confronted with his own healthy and positive behavior and motivated to see himself as someone who, despite limitations, is mature and takes the possessions and interests of others into account (as opposed to being a thief and/or taking advantage of others). The next step would be to seriously debate with the client and discuss behavior that is inappropriate and may call for sanctions such as fines or prison sentences, and offering alternatives instead. If these interventions/forms of persuasion are not beneficial, (then) care professionals can alert other institutions such as the police or justice system. However, whether or not this effectively changes the clients' actions remains questionable. Often, the involvement of police will actually lead to (increased) resistance on the part of the client. In that case it may be advisable to explore other options (such as alerting social work or people from the healthy environment of the client). The tendency not to rush to the police can (easily) be defended because an exaggerated intervention may result in negative reactions from the client and thus damage the basis of trust that is essential for a good professional relationship. Nevertheless, in some cases there is no other way as the client systematically ignores well-intended advices. In a selected group of patients clarity and an active stance can help to break the cycle of negativity.

5. Carefulness

From the viewpoint of care ethics, action may indeed be indicated when looking out for the client's autonomy. This does not purport that every form of intervention is always justified. First of all, the intervention should have a result. Will the intervention modify the client's behavior, end the criminal activities, and help the client to find pursuits that are more compatible with his abilities? An ineffective intervention will inevitably be problematical. Secondly, the intervention should be appropriate, and specifically not more grave than necessary. For example, a minor incidental offense demands a straightforward but small correction and some form of agreement to prevent repetition. When a client is structurally involved in unlawful activity the care professional may consider applying some restrictions (for instance taking away certain privileges) or alerting other institutions and authorities. To be able to answer these questions it is vital to pay attention to the client's reactions. Herein, observation and communication are essential.

A care ethical attitude requires the willingness of care professionals to take on responsibilities, but also to be open to the reactions of the recipient/client, and, if necessary, to amend their own opinions about giving good care. Openness demands that one does not ignore possible negative reactions from others. Conversely, it also does not mean that every negative response or refusal should be considered to be just. To be able to modify one's opinions there needs to be trust and a firm, but not inflexible belief in one's own standpoints and perceptions. Adequate help constitutes the ability to find a middle ground between determination and resoluteness on the one hand and acquiescence and flexibility on the other hand. Adhering too strongly to your own beliefs impairs the capability to hear the negative reactions of others. However, following every suggestion of another person could result in a decreased value of one's own ideas and beliefs. It also makes one incredible and untrustworthy. According to Aristotle, the capability to determine the right means and course of action in a given situation is characteristic of wise and intelligent people (Widdershoven, 2000). The type of wisdom that is of concern here is primarily practical in nature. This is therefore called practical wisdom. Rather than pointing out the middle ground through reasoning, what matters is demonstrating this through (one's) actions, situated in time, place, and circumstances.

Practical wisdom implies one is capable of shaping behavior in such a way that extremes are avoided. In care, this means that care professionals know when and what kind of coercive measures are indicated and appropriate in the situation, but also when they should hold back (in these) and find alternatives which are less restricting. Only on the basis of practical wisdom can you responsibly realize the interventions that Moody (1992) proposes. After all, the question of whether a certain intervention is justified in the situation and whether or not it is too severe or too light keeps repeating itself. This does not only include the consideration of whether the type of intervention will be successful or not, but also whether the intervention is appropriate in answering the question of what good care is and how this can be answered in cooperation.

Discussing incidents after they have occurred with care professionals, clients, and other involved parties is part of good care. This enables the care professional to calmly explain the measures that were taken, why they were taken, the dilemma's experienced, the emotions and feelings the intervention evoked among professionals, how this affected the client, and whether he understood the care professional's motivation. Evaluation offers the client the chance to share experiences and feelings, to ask questions and raise concerns. It does not occur often, but the participants generally appreciate talking about such matters. It helps the client to hear that the care professional saw no other way out and also felt concerned and bothered by it. Voicing these feelings promotes understanding (Widdershoven & Berghmans, 2005). Not only can such an evaluation be an opportunity to exchange views on the situation and express emotions and experiences (often feelings of powerlessness on the side of the care professionals, and anger and resentment on the part of the clients), but it will also serve to advance learning and generate ideas how to prevent crises in the near future. Why was an intervention needed? Could looking out for certain behaviors earlier on have prevented the intervention? What does this mean for the future? Based on the findings it is frequently possible to create early intervention plans and make appointments with the client. In this way communication, evaluation, and prevention go hand in hand (Abma et al., 2005).

6. Conclusion

Societies are less tolerant toward criminal and strange behavior of certain patient populations than several decades ago. It is therefore nowadays more or less expected that care professionals report certain behaviors to each other, the police or the authorities. This article raised the issue how to deal with these new sets of responsibilities from a care ethics perspective.

Commonly care professionals tend to not to interfere in the lives and privacy of clients referring to the value of autonomy. Respect for autonomy can, however, be explicated in a number of ways. From the viewpoint of negative freedom/liberty one should give people the space and opportunity to make their own decisions and not interfere. Here, the contents of their choices are irrelevant. People are seen as individuals who, ideally, live their lives independently of each other. From a care ethical perspective, the idea of positive freedom/liberty is propagated. People are free when they are allowed to develop and are able to handle the situation they are in. This requires an inter-subjective context of care and support. Giving direction to his own life does not mean that a client can do whatever he wants without hindrance or impediment. It does mean that a client is able to structure and build his own life supported by the attention and involvement of others and that he learns how to handle his disabilities and cope with his limitations.

Based on the care ethical view of autonomy it would be useful if care professionals keep each other informed of problematic behavior in their clients. Alerting police or the justice system may also be indicated. Such forms of intervention should, however, be subject to certain requirements. Firstly, all parties involved should aim to enhance the autonomy of the client. This will enable him to get more control over his situation. Secondly, the least severe intervention should be employed. Stimulation and persuasion are preferable to coercion. Lastly, the intervention should be evaluated with all parties.

7. References

Abma, T.A., G.A.M. Widdershoven e.a. (red.) *Dwang en drang in de psychiatrie, De kwaliteit van vrijheidsbeperkende maatregelen* Utrecht, Lemma, 2005.

Agich, G.J. *Autonomy and long-term care*Oxford: Oxford University Press, 1993.

Beauchamp, T.L., J.F.Childress*Principles of biomedical ethics* Oxford: Oxford University Press, 1994.

Berlin, I. *Four essays on liberty* Oxford, Oxford University Press, 1969.

Dworkin, G. *The theory and practice of autonomy* New York, Cambridge University Press, 1988.

Emanuel, E.J., L.L. Emanuel Four models of the Physician-patient Relationship JAMA, April 22/29, 267(16): 2221-2226, 1992.

Guadagnoli, E., P. Ward, Patient Participation in Decision-Making *Social Science and Medicine*, 47(3): 329-339, 1988.

Mackenzie, C., N. Stoljar (red.) *Relational Autonomy* Oxford, Oxford University Press, 2000.

Mill, J.S. *On liberty* Harmondsworth, Penguin, 1859.

Moody, H.R. *Ethics in an aging society* Baltimore, Johns Hopkins University Press, 1992.

Oeseburg, B., T.A. Abma Care as a mutual endeavour, Medicine, Health Care and Philosophy, 9: 349-357, 2006.

Ricoeur, P. *Oneself as Another.* (transl. from french by Blamey K ; original title : Soi-même, comme un autre). Chicago/London:The University of Chicago Press, 1992.

Thorne, S., B. Paterson Shifting Images of Chronic Illness *Journal of Nursing Scholarship*, 30(2), 173-178, 1998.

Tronto, J. *Moral Boundaries* New York: Routledge, 1993.

Verkerk, M.A. The Care Perspective and Autonomy Medicine, *Health Care and Philosophy*, 4(3), 2001 (a), pp. 289-294.

Verkerk, M.A.Over drang als goed zorgen: een zorgethische benadering. *Tijdschrift voor Geneeskunde en Ethiek*, 11e jaargang, nr. 4, 2001 (b), pp. 101-106.

Verkerk, M.A. Zorgethiek: naar een geografie van verantwoordelijkheden In: Manschot H.A.M.. H van Dartel (red.), *In gesprek over goede zorg*, Amsterdam/Meppel, Uitgeverij Boom, 2003, pp. 177-190.

Widdershoven, G. *Ethiek in de kliniek* Amsterdam/Meppel, Uitgeverij Boom, 2000.

Widdershoven, G., R. Berghmans Dwang en drang vanuit een ethisch perspectief In: Abma, T.A., G.A.M. Widdershoven e.a. (red.), *Dwang en drang in de psychiatrie, De kwaliteit van vrijheidsbeperkende maatregelen*, Utrecht, Lemma, 2005, pp. 44-54.

4

Bioethics and Modern Technology: Reasons of Concern

Rolando V. Jiménez-Domínguez and Onofre Rojo-Asenjo
Centro de Investigaciones Económicas, Administrativas y Sociales (CIECAS) del Instituto Politécnico Nacional México

1. Introduction

Today's world technology, more than any other human activity, is transforming our lives, our habits and life styles, the ways human beings relate to each other; it creates our material wealth and the bases of our progress and modern civilization, that is to say, our economy. It is not improper to say, in a word, that modern technology makes our world. However, this abundant source of benefits is not free from inconveniences, some of which may seriously endanger fundamental aspects of nature and human life [Arthur, 2009; Kelly, 2010].

Thanks to the scientific and technological advance during the last 150 years, infant mortality has been enormously reduced and life expectancy of people has almost doubled. We have found effective treatments for many diseases which were before mortal, and the hygiene conditions of most of the world population have been considerably improved. This has brought at the same time a huge growth of this population, which has grown from one thousand million at the middle of the nineteen century to almost seven thousand million beginning the second decade of the XXI century, what is giving rise to serious difficulties in providing adequate living conditions for every human being. Antibiotics have saved countless lives while making it possible for new and incredibly virulent bacteria to evolve. The convenience of e-mail turns into communication overload; face to face contacts are being substituted by screen to screen communications. Even our most publicized inventions can turn on us. Contradiction seems to be the name of the game: the past century was history's deadliest, in terms of humanity's technological capacity for organized violence. And yet life expectancies in the industrialized world, as mentioned, rose to approach eighty years.

Nuclear energy developments have encountered useful applications in the generation of electric energy for many regions of the earth, as well as applications in the medical fields, but at the same time have created the possibility of massive annihilation of all kinds of creatures, including the human, and the destruction of ecology at large. Genetic manipulation is associated with our hopes for attainment of a life free of diseases and other sufferings, but it is also opening possibilities of interventions in the natural evolution processes of living organisms with unpredictable consequences. Any prediction based on the genetic determinism is nowadays strongly questioned, since there are no reasons to accept that the characteristics of a living organism are only determined by their genes [Ho, 1998].

Experience teaches us that every good outcome from the scientific-technological progress is always accompanied by reasons of concern; there is an implicit contradiction in the progress: every result can be both beneficial and harmful, without the possibility to separate these characteristics; the old dilemma of good and wrong. But in this dilemma there is some degree of relativism which makes even more difficult the decision; sometimes what is good or wrong depends on the decisions-taker point of view. A dam which is used to provide water and electricity for a city is certainly good, from the point of view of those who receive this benefit. But perhaps the same dam required the displacement of thousands of people and destroys an ecosystem, and from this point of view is bad. The important questions are then: Who chooses? Who wins? Who loses? [Lightman et al., 2003].

If we consider some other recent technological advances, like genetics engineering (genetic manipulation, cloning, assisted reproduction), neurotechnologies, etc., we have to deal with more complex situations to decide between what is more convenient to be done and what we must avoid in order to prevent severe damages to human life and values. Thus we can convince ourselves that technology, which up to now we have seen as the best instrument man has to improve his life, can be at the same time a powerful means for transforming his nature and values in a way that is unacceptable for some of us up to the point of rising the question if man will be able to survive his ingenuity and creativity.

In this work we shall be concerned with the implications that the development of modern technology has on human values, and in this respect we shall consider some specific situations which are already giving rise to ethical dilemmas requiring urgent answers. Next we review some fundamental concepts related to the problems at hand. In the last part of the work we shall discuss the topic of social responsibility and the role the whole society can play in search of solutions to the ethical problems posed by the technological advance. We end up looking for rational arguments to support an optimistic vision of our future technological development.

2. The impacts of technological development

The technological development occurred during the past 100 years has provided the infrastructure needed to revolutionize the study, the knowledge and manipulation of life, including human life itself; it has changed and accelerated communications among persons and countries; it has altered the "goods and services" production systems while creating new and threatening problems which place humanity on the brink of extinction … or happiness! Today, starting the second decade of XXI century, the topics of our times are in connection with the most advanced technologies, which open for almost everybody the possibility of creative or destructive actions surpassing our most audacious speculations about future, not imagined before.

In 1976, after the discovery of the recombinant DNA techniques and the potential risks due to its use which allow, in principle, the design of new living organisms with characteristics selected at will by the experimenter, the United States National Institute of Health (NIH) established the conditions required to carry out these kind of experiments, fixing the security levels corresponding to the varying characteristics of creatures under study. Nevertheless, some local authorities rejected these rules of national security and asked for the open discussion of these issues in committees designed *ad hoc*, in order to guarantee the free participation of all interested persons and avoid any alleged manipulation; in this way they expected to dissipate fears and distrustful thinking of the people. These committees would study all risks involved and propose recommendations about the convenience or inconvenience of authorizing experiments on recombinant DNA and, in case of approval, in what conditions. The deliberations were carried out but neither definitive answers nor compulsory measures were obtained, and much less agreement in all respects; but the proposed questions and the individually adopted answers opened the way for new approaches to the problem, based on questions like: Is it possible to separate the ethical issues associated with the experiments from those related to its applications? Is it possible to separate the creation of new forms of plants or microbes from the creation of new types of human beings? And assuming that genetic manipulation of human beings is possible in practice, what would be the prevailing ethics: that of human fraternity or the ethics based on the right to be different? Is commercial exploitation of recombinant DNA ethically different from commercial exploitation of other techniques? Does gene implantation from higher to lower level organisms represent a dangerous transgression of the barriers between biological species? Have we the right to interfere in the natural evolutive processes without knowing the possible outcomes? ... etc. [Dyson, 1993].

In a different field of knowledge, the development of information technologies and social networks (Internet, Facebook, etc.) are drastically changing the political order and the traditional courses of action and modalities of citizen's participation. It is not possible to predict the future course of events, but recent cases like those of Tunisia and Egypt could be replicated and perhaps the revolutions of XXI century will be done not with arms but with cell phones and will be transmitted by Internet, since these media provide the means to express the desires for freedom and justice that sometimes official censorship restricts through public broadcasting media and printed press. These are revolutions without visible leaders but with visible technology that connects people and enables common citizens to express their dreams and desires through message texts and twits.

This sudden change in the ways people are connected comes together with another revolution that takes place within us, since cell phones enable us to be closer to distant persons and more distant of those who are near. If we observe any line of persons waiting for bus, show or restaurant, we notice that people are talking by phone with somebody far away instead of talking with their neighbors in the same cue. This occurs so frequently that answering a phone call and talking with distant persons in the middle of a social gathering is not anymore considered as impolite. Our values in this respect have changed.

These facts convince us that social values change quickly as a result of the new communication technologies, and this is because eight of every ten inhabitants of this planet have access to a cell phone, what amounts to 5,300 million according to the International Telecommunications Union belonging to the United Nations. There exist today two thousand million with access to Internet and this number is growing every day. Modern communications not only put down tyrants; they also change our habits and customs.

Our age is characterized by the success of physical technologies, in what has been termed Second Industrial Revolution: automatism, space conquest, atomic bomb, genetic medicine, cloning, etc. We can say without arrogance that human life has suffered more changes in the last decades than in any other earlier period of history [Drucker, 2011]. But at the same time, progress has brought worries and dire visions in connection with the same aspects that were improved: the threat of a thermonuclear war, the population explosion due to the increase in life expectancy, etc. This is the price we have to pay for living in a cybernetic society. Present day societies oscillates between hopes and satisfaction, on one hand, and fears on the other;

technological marvels in medicine and urban life are counterbalanced by the real possibilities of nuclear destruction. Ecology has been seriously affected by what we have called technical progress, and if we do not change our concept of good living standard to make it more sustainable our cybernetic society will be on the verge of collapse.

History has shown that whenever humanity reached any limit situation it was necessary to build new social structures and review current moral values and its hierarchy in such a way that survival could be assured. This does not imply the construction of a completely new morality, but the adaptation of what we can consider human intrinsic values to the new situation. Today we are confronted for the first time in history with situations that need special attention: some of the new artifacts emerging from the new technologies have such a destructive potential that can destroy all life in extended regions of the planet, and can be used by a single person. The only consideration of this possibility is terrifying. The problem is not that today's scientific-technological development is more advanced than before, but that the traditional role of mere mediators played by science and technology is not in correspondence with the role effectively played by them today. Modern science and technology are not only intermediaries between human life and nature. They are new ways of living and thinking; even our art and philosophy have changed in accordance. These are the main reasons to consider the issue of human values as a priority, and also the underlying arguments for the creation of the field of bioethics in connection with technology. This is the idea behind the expression "bioethics is a bridge to the future", which its founder [Potter, 1988] used as the title of one of his books, as we shall see in what follows.

3. The ethical dimension of development. The emergence of bioethics

In the new technology-oriented society the interactions between humanistic and scientific-technological concepts are so frequent and intense that those concepts will necessarily converge and tend towards common meanings. This understanding can be achieved through bioethics, which harmonizes the values shared by society and the challenges arising from the technical development. Some of the promises that technology offers exceed our most audacious Utopias. Newspapers daily reports on new scientific findings and new technological developments rise ideological confrontations whose base is essentially an ethical debate. Many of these confrontations are the result of ideological or economic struggles in search of power, but even in those cases there is a common background with strong bioethical implications. There was a time in which science could be considered as pure thinking and curiosity, and the phrase "thought is not delinquent" was used to separate it from any axiological consideration to avoid "inquisitions and faith acts". We cannot hold this position anymore, as has been exemplified by the famous exclamation of J. Robert Oppenheimer when he declared, as the main scientist in charge, after witnessing the first successful explosion of the newly constructed atomic bomb at Alamo Gordo, New Mexico: "In a profound sense which cannot be distorted by any malicious interpretation, we, the scientists, have known the sin" [Schweber, 2000]. The underlying meaning of this sentence was not that the scientific community had lost innocence and was thrown off paradise, but that the binomial science-technology (not necessarily in that order) leads to a new conception of man and the world. Science and technology are not axiologically neutral, they transform and determine the human experience and even the relation between human beings and the world, through the ways humans understand and handle the world itself: if man is conceived as a programmable machine, this necessarily influences all decisions about people. These considerations lead to bioethics as a discipline constructed on the facts that have been objectively established through a dialogue between different visions of the world and man, in order to make sense of that world and the man who inhabits it.

The birth of modern bioethics is historically linked to some abuses in scientific research with human beings, carried out in the past century, especially those performed in Germany during the Second World War. Nuremberg trials exposed these facts so they were generally known the world over. Nuremberg Code, published in 1946, paved the way for the establishment of norms to protect the integrity of human subjects in biomedical experimentation. The main criteria to achieve these goals include safeguards like the previous informed consent, the subject's liberty to abandon the experiment at any time, and the experimenter's ethics. The first evaluation of a biomedical research protocol was carried out in 1953, when the NIH of the United States applied these criteria to every research with human subjects intended to be done in its Betheshda Hospital. This same spirit and normativity appear later, in 1964, as agreements of the World Medical Association (Helsinki Declaration), which recommends the integration of committees, independent of researchers and sponsors, aimed to project evaluation from the ethical point of view. It is in the field of genetics where these moral issues are more clearly perceived. Experimentation with human subjects is necessary even in those cases where genetic diagnosis and associated therapies can be tested and verified in animals, since that is the only way to guarantee that the results will be equally successful when applied to humans. Today we know that those results cannot be translated directly, without further tests, from animals to humans, because each biological entity has peculiar responses to the same conditions; the environmental conditions can affect the response too, even within the same species: the immunological response against treatments or invading agents is not the same in all human beings. This fact makes it necessary to test vaccines directly on the risk population before its general application, and this implies experimentation with human beings. Decisions in connection to these problems can only be taken after a careful analysis and discussion in a plural committee, in which human dignity, liberty and benefit can be preserved without stigmatization or discrimination. Thus, bioethics is the instrument needed to solve the problems derived from the moral dilemmas due to the new technologies, which cannot be solved by traditional ethics.

Bioethics emerges as a discipline at the beginning of the decade of 1970, and Van Rensselaer Potter [1988], who is considered its founder, states it in a rather ample sense: to discuss what it is ethically right or wrong about man's increasing capacity of intervention on nature, and the possibility that this intervention endangers life on earth [Ferrer & Álvarez, 2003]. Nevertheless, the field of bioethics is frequently restricted to the study of the moral implications and consequences arising from the medical practice. However, it is not less important that bioethical studies consider also those aspects of scientific-technological developments that have an impact on human life, both social and individually.

It must be taken into account that ethics is not a set of simple and clearly defined norms that have no exceptions and apply automatically to any concrete situation; if this were the case, it would be useless in complex or uncertain situations. Ethics is neither a set of ideals, admirable but unrealistic, that can never be reached. Instead, ethics is composed by norms and principles that have to be harmonized and conjugated with other norms and principles, and with the data from reality, giving rise to objective axiological conflicts which must be solved to distinguish the right actions and to justify them. It cannot be completely objective, due to its relation with culture, so moral absolutism must be discarded; it cannot be either totally subjective (moral relativism). But the survival of any society needs at least a set of minimum moral agreements, and then we are led to the question: is there an intermediate way between moral absolutism and moral relativism? If the objective-relative structure of moral life is admitted, then this would be the answer; there are moral values which are not created by the moral subject, but exist in the things themselves.

Humankind is not only interested in assuring its future survival and welfare, but wants to be ruled with criteria based on rights and justice, preserving his dignity and avoiding the rule of those who have only the power. This needs the establishment of a living-together culture. It is very important to understand that technology can help human beings not only in the construction of their future material world but also to transform human reality. In this historical moment, science and technology are not only means to provide goods and services but are also very effective instruments to modulate the people´s substrate which we call culture. More than the economic relationships, science and technology transform the nature of the relationships among the peoples by transforming their vision of reality as a consequence of the use of new knowledge and techniques.

The factors that define a culture, like historical identity and connections with neighbors and other cultures, will be transformed as a consequence of the technological advance. Globalization, a phenomenon partially due to technical progress, is making almost impossible for a civilization to remain isolated from the rest of the world. Even in the most isolated places, people's culture is affected by technological change, and that includes also the field of people's values.

There exist two factors that make our civilization unique in comparison of those already disappeared: one is the technological development, which makes possible to control nature to an extend never before attained, opening possibilities to alleviate hunger, diseases, and super population; the other one, which can be considered a consequence of the first, is the global character of our civilization.

Modern technological civilization is not the privilege of groups or particular nations; is open to every human being belonging to any culture, race or religious affiliation. The values and creativity in this civilization are being transformed and adapted to the material changes, in such a way than if the fights for power in this critical phase of world situation (which confront us with serious risks of a universal atomic devastation) are finally overcome, the differences between East and West could become insignificant due to the similarities of material cultures, that in the long term will prove to be stronger than ideological differences.

The strong attraction that comes out the technological progress, and its possibilities for attaining rapid results, lead us to consider the discussion about values as a time loss, as well as the debates about possible catastrophic results. Reason is left apart, as a measure of moral value and norm to choose between right and wrong, just or unfair, and it is replaced by a risk-benefit assessment, which gives rise to disagreements and difficulties leading to unending debates in bioethics committees, which will be analyzed later.

In order to establish a social compromise with bioethical characteristics to face the challenges posed by techno-scientific innovations and impacts due to globalization processes, we need to carry out a careful discussion about the limits of science and technology and our possibilities and constraints as a human group, contrasting the empirical and/or phenomenological reality with theoretical or operational positions that involve ethical demands. Thus, theoretical studies cannot be restricted to the construction of interpretative systems, but must also include the ways to face them: aside of interpreting and understanding the structure and dynamics of the techno-scientific innovation processes, their stabilization and transformation, we need to assess the impact, consequences and ways of intervention in those processes. Otherwise our task will remain unaccomplished. Then, in order to fully understand the ethical dimension of technological progress, we need to know how technology emerges, the mechanisms by which it evolves and how it is connected to innovation. These are topics not completely explored, but there are some interesting works that have initiated this journey [Arthur, 2009; Kelly, 2010]] that eventually will produce a theory of technology.

3.1 The case of genetically manipulated varieties. Transgenics

The use of recombining DNA in agriculture for farming improvement or plague elimination must be done through experimentation in the natural environment, in order to produce those genetically modified varieties and leave them free. But this kind of experiments is strongly opposed by irrational groups that monopolize the right of defending the planet. This is the real problem with transgenics. The groups opposing experiments on genetically modified varieties are frequently aggressive and stubbornly closed to arguments presented by other groups in favor of experimentation; the dialogue is almost impossible. Prudence is good but not extreme positions opposing any testimony. According to Matt Ridley, British zoologist, "After consuming more than a trillion meals prepared with transgenic food there are no reports about any diseases caused by genetically manipulated plants" [Ridley, 2010]. A similar statement was published by the United Nations: there is no evidence, up to now, about harmful effects due to the genetically modified varieties present in human food supplies. The gene transfer between different species, crossing the barriers which separate them, is not a natural process; in consequence, wheat, the most cultivated plant in the world is an unnatural polyploid mixture of at least three wild wheat plants. Transgenics could be a solution to the problem of increasing agriculture production to meet the continuous population growth.

However, it is very important to proceed cautiously, because according to genetics engineering specialist Mae-Wan Ho [1998]: techniques for genetic recombination are designed specifically for gene transfer horizontally between species that do not cross reproduce, and can destroy the defensive mechanisms of mixed species. If we eliminate the natural biological diversity, which is the result of a very long evolutive process, any plague could destroy in a very short time all members of given species. These techniques are also used by an industry that sells illusions for the people (cancer medicines, baby design, cloning, and other means to reach immortality). This industry is patenting almost everything and converting in merchandise the parts of every living creature, including man itself. When experiments respond to market's interest we have to proceed carefully.

It is now possible for a child to have up to five parents: the egg donor, the sperm donor, the surrogate mother who carries the baby and the couple who raises the child. Cloning is also becoming just another form of assisted reproduction; then, on the other hand, a child might have just one parent. Consequently, the notion of family is changing and even concepts like "normality" have to be adjusted to the new possibilities. It is possible to generate a genetic profile of a child before birth; twelve percent of potential parents say they would abort a fetus with a genetic propensity toward obesity. The designing of children is occurring subtly, as a result of individual choices in an open market. There is a strong controversy over human embryonic stem-cell research. Although the applications of stem cells remain on a speculative base, a marked debate has taken place in connection with the morality of destroying embryos for research. To portray the struggle as one of rationality versus the forces of darkness seems to be very simplistic. This is why we need additional research, avoid radical positions, and invite people to participate in all decisions that affect society.

3.2 Neurosciences

The development of new technologies for studying the human brain has open countless possibilities for understanding consciousness and mental functions, but at the same time this techniques are giving rise to problems and questionings for which it is important to take into account the moral common sense, the values, and all ethical considerations.

The ethical issues raised by advances in neuroscience are with us already. These issues overlap and even outflank the ones raised by genetic engineering. Changing the brain, with or without gene alteration, speaks of what it means to be human. Drugs or magnetic fields that modulate the cognition may bend the very definition of what we are.

What kinds of safeguards are needed if a machine can read your thoughts? Will cognition enhancers exacerbate differences between rich and poor? Or will social diversity become a status of historical artifact? Is technology a means for reducing marginality of poor people or on the contrary, is contributing to increase the gap between the very rich and the very poor?

The technologies of mind and brain are different from those related to genomics and other biomedical fields in an important respect: as most scientists and ethicists acknowledge, the essence of what we are is not all in our genes.

Can neurosciences provide some answers to the ethical issues raised by its advances? In this respect it is of interest for our purposes to bring about the psychobiological studies done in Harvard University under the directorship of Dr. Marc D. Hauser. In his book *Moral Minds* [2006], Dr. Hauser establishes the existence of a basic moral sentiment or feeling, resulting from human evolution, which acts as a survival mechanism: the fact that human societies share almost universally some basic norms or guidelines for action, suggests that there is a general moral structure emerging from the human neural constitution that is still evolving, not yet in its final form. Then, the resulting human intelligence is also in a changing process, what makes it different from artificial intelligence, which up to now only evolves by external influence or innovations.

The power of these new "neurotechnologies" associated with neurosciences and psychobiology is astonishing; almost daily one can learn about new gadgets able to read face expressions of people, watching and correcting their movements, etc. It would seem that human autonomy is now in danger. Nevertheless, we must be prudent in the handling of these achievements and use them for improving our life and live together. Or, as Winner [2008] expresses:

> *"If we realize up to what point our lives are molded by modern technology interconnected systems and how intense is this influence, accept its authority and participate in its functioning, we will start to understand that we already became members of a new order in mankind history"*

In the second decade of past century Spanish philosopher José Ortega y Gasset [2005] proposed as the topic of our times the role scientific development was playing in social changes and cultural perspectives at the time; his vision was optimistic, trustful on the progress and having science as modern panacea. Many things has happened since, and after the two world wars and the menace of massive annihilation, that confidence has been lessened and replaced by an almost cosmic pessimism that associates progress and development with risk, uncertainty and anguish.

Today the success of a technology can be measured by its beneficial effects on human life. According to this, the most successful of all modern technologies are those associated to life and health. We have already mentioned transgenics, but there are many more:

> *"Man feels now able to create biological species and this is serious; the production of biological systems that did not exist since the dawn of times opens possibilities of creating chimeras, what implies the rupture of the natural species concept" [Laín-Entralgo, 1994].*

This all leads to a reconsideration of operating laws and new approaches to moral acts. The technological change is also influencing some other concepts like that of human generation. In the first half of XX Century was still valid Ortega y Gasset's [2005] vision expressed as:

> *"... Life changes but not in a continuous way. It has some stability, that is: life style lasts certain time. Life is based on opinions, valuations, imperatives, characterized by its acceptance and validity, prevailing in the society. They are imposed to any individual, independently of its free acceptance. The operating time of this norms and rules system is more or less coincident with fifteen years. Thus, a generation is a zone of fifteen years during which life is almost uniform. This would be the authentic unit in history´s chronology."*

Compare this vision with today´s situation in which the acceleration of social development dynamics can change in few months, and a system of gadgets and its use is imposed to any individual, accepted or not. Since the beginnings of radio, passing through TV, Internet, Facebook and Twitter, the technological advances define what a generation is, with its own uses and customs, establishing a new unit for history´s chronology with global character, overcoming sometimes centuries of differences between countries. Tunisia´s last revolt has much to do with the existence of social networks, which united people in a common wish to put down a dictatorship of more than 20 years.

The power and potential force that technology endows to governments and enterprises makes critical the consideration of human rights that should not be violated. After a terrific world war which seemed to vanish all rules between peoples for living together, it was necessary the creation of an international instrument to protect humankind against the unlimited power of the state governments. This was the birth of the Universal Chart of Human Rights, and the origin of several movements questioning, at citizen´s level, the validity of certain actions that could be justified from the scientific and technical points of view but were inconsistent with human dignity and security. These movements defended the right of people to previous informed consent and participation in all decisions affecting them, not to be used as experiment subjects only. Bioethics movement was born this way.

4. The problem of values

Values are the qualities associated with some realities that are considered good and appreciated; they posses polarity and hierarchy. Thus, values can be considered positive and negative, major and minor, but without price in money. Human values as liberty, dignity, autonomy, cannot be purchased or traded, in spite that in past times (and perhaps even today) they were purchased as in the case of slaves paying for their liberty or freedom. Technology has induced changes in society's structure; however, it cannot make *tabula rasa* with human values, since these are perhaps printed somehow in the specie's neuronal structure, as we mentioned before in relation with neurosciences [Churchland, 2011]. They must be adapted to a new reality and establish a balance (not in financial terms) between what is obtained and what is lost, with full knowledge of advantages and disadvantages and with previous informed consent of individuals. Every technical advance means change (innovation), but the essence of human values must be preserved. Technology not necessarily produces a sick society, as some voices claim, if we temperate its consequences by harmonizing innovations with human values.

Ethics of technology is not anymore what Aristotle wanted: the *recta ratio factibilium* [Laín-Entralgo, 1994], since technological possibilities today raise situations whose solutions must be based on an assessment of the results and consequences derived from the actions carried out. Today's technology is having a marked exponential growth [Kurzweil, 2005] but few opportunities to answer some questions regarding its social consequences and impacts on human values. A neat and honest consideration of these answers leads frequently to a conflict between final purposes and values, and if there exist conflict between purposes and values it becomes very important to proceed cautiously in establishing priorities. We are now facing situations which can imply the massive destruction of species, including ours; we can create instruments that can attempt against human dignity and individual privacy (informatics technologies of "hacking" or electronic information robbery). What to do? Stop technical advances? It would not be feasible. It is better to initiate a serious reflection to determine if all what is possible should be done or not and establish a balance "between what should be done and what should not be done within what can be done". Ethics would be then the right reason (*recta ratio*) in this discussion, which is achieved not by means of an individual reflection but by interdisciplinary deliberation within a group honestly interested in encountering answers and free of constraints or compromises.

Freeman Dyson, a renowned scientist, was invited by Princeton's Major to become a member of a group integrated by eleven persons to deliberate about citizen's distrust on recombinant DNA experiments. The group was composed by two physicians, three writers, three scientists, a teacher, a Presbyterian minister, and a housekeeper. Later F. Dyson reported his experience during the deliberations and pointed out that: "The first lesson we learned was about the importance of listening. The only way to eliminate distrust is to hear those persons who are in disagreement with us and convince them to hear patiently the arguments presented by their critics." [Dyson, 1993].

Each controversial topic could be carefully discussed attending every possible point of view; the result could be at least to create in the experimenters or decision takers a cautious attitude that prevents monstrosities derived from the unrestricted confidence on science and its applications, as sometimes occurred in the past.

The quality of a society is not measured by the amount of knowledge it handles, but by the values applied in the use of that knowledge; the problems generated by the uses of technology should be analyzed under this criterion. Unfortunately, as an almost general result we could state that new technologies have contributed to enhance the gap between the rich, technically prepared and informatized, and the poor deprived of computers and technically illiterate; they have made possible the emergence of a society that does not allow uneducated young people to find an honorable way of living, but at the same time creates many opportunities for those with easy access to the world of high technology.

5. Social participation, not only the experts

Once a complex technology has been extensively diffused and adopted, it is extremely difficult to replace it, or even restrict or reorient it. Powerful economic interests and social inertia that opposes changes make things happen this way. Some common examples are the automobile and the TV: any attempt to restrict or alter the modalities of their use will find strong opposition from large sectors of society. Then, the proper selection of the technologies that will be adopted by society requires our participation from the beginning, in order to evaluate the pertinence and possible benefits or disadvantages that will result from its adoption. This participation requires, of course, the most complete information available and the discussion. Scientists or technology experts tend to ignore or undervalue opinions coming from unprofessional persons when the discussion is about complex technological developments, but they forget that research and experiments are paid by society and that is society at large who faces the consequences when something goes wrong and results are not as good as expected.

Another important fact that we must take into account is that recently adopted technologies are not always available to all sectors of the society, so its benefits are restricted to small groups. For example, neurotechnologies to enhance memory or learning capacities of people could be inaccessible to large sectors of the society, by economic or political reasons. In that case, would not these technologies increase the gap between the rich and the poor? ... Or between developed and underdeveloped countries? Is it fair that only the educated people of a country can have access to the best opportunities and living standards? Is it acceptable that marginal groups of society would be condemned to hunger or unemployment?

If technology establishes the limits of what we can do and ethics the limits of what we should do, it seems reasonable to start a dialogue between them. The best and simplest way to establish such a dialogue is through a committee integrated in the most plural way, where all social actors are represented, not only the experts. Because, finally: Who is really an expert when we are trying to foresee the future development of an emergent technology? Take, for example, the research on genomics and human reproduction techniques by genetic manipulations with the use of stem cells; this has been a polemic field from the very beginning, in spite of the fact that possible applications are still of an essentially speculative character. Could these research areas with a high potential to transform society proceed independently from public deliberation?

On the other hand, the technological products that can affect human life operate in an empty legal context, with no governmental regulations or proper social surveillance. Social groups oscillate between absolute apathy and irrational emotivity, opposing all changes and progress. This is why the discussion of these topics becomes so important when it is carried out in the core of a well-informed society. The ethical consequence of technological progress is a concern not only of the experts but of all affected people.

Another issue in which the ethical considerations are of primary importance is that of global warming and climate change. This is mainly due to the CO_2 emissions produced in the industrialized countries, but the victims of the more severe damages are those living in the poorest countries; they lose their homes, crops and lands when their regions are hit by hurricanes or droughts. A global policy to control greenhouse gas emissions can come only from a free an independent ethics-based decision taken by the major countries, since no other mechanism is at hand to press those countries to do so. In this broader stage, it is very desirable that more and more countries participate in the design of the ethical frames that will regulate human relationships in the coming years. This task should not be accomplished exclusively by the technologically advanced nations; it would be a fundamental contradiction.

5.1 Bioethics committees

Our modern societies are eager to receive the benefits from the scientific-technological development, but without paying a high price for mistakes and its consequences that frequently come together with some researches. This makes it necessary to supervise openly the interdisciplinary committees that will give suggestions and recommendations about research activities and proposals, looking to preserve individual liberty, dignity, and benefit. Conflicts arising from these discussions, which are not easy to overcome, have to be solved at a final executive level.

The commission mentioned by F. Dyson [1993] is a variation of the Institutional Review Boards (IRB) which the Department of Health and Human Services (DHHS) of the United States in its Regulations for the Protection of Human Subjects established in 1991:

> *"a) Each IRB shall have at least five members with varying backgrounds to promote adequate and complete review of research activities commonly conducted by the institution. The IRB shall be sufficiently qualified through the experience and expertise of its members and the diversity of the members, including race, gender and cultural backgrounds and sensitivity in such issues as community attitudes, to promote respect for its advice and counsel. Each IRB shall include at least one member whose primary concerns are in nonscientific areas."*

Those committees are deliberating organisms that make careful and complete considerations about the advantages and disadvantages of any decision prior to its adoption, with votes fully supported before emitted. This deliberation about situations that are partially known but whose effects or consequences are not clear or predetermined, is carried out by exchanging personal arguments and points of view in a dialogical process whose only purpose is to find the truth, leaving apart any dogmatic position. This is the philosophy that should be applied to the analysis of the technological research that can affect human life and values. The work of a bioethics committee, according to Diego Gracia, a Spanish expert in these topics [cited by Martínez, 2003, p. 70], must proceed in the following way:

1. Identify the problem
2. Analyze the "relevant facts" with the highest possible precision
3. Identify the involved values
4. Identify conflicting values
5. Identify the fundamental or most important conflict between values
6. Deliberate about possible courses of action
7. Deliberate about the course of action that optimizes conflicting values. Determine the most convenient course of action
8. Deliberate about agreement between most convenient course of action and culture
9. Take a final decision.
10. Check the legal or illegal aspects of this final decision.

Today these Bioethics Committees are integrated and in operation in almost all hospitals and medical research centers around the world, and had been taken as models for the integration and operation of similar committees in other fields of scientific research.

6. Are there any bases for rational optimism?

The answer to this question depends on the point of view we adopt or the group we belong to, since there are at least two possible positions in relation to the future evolution of technology: the position of those who do not accept that technological development could change the nature of human beings and the traditional values of humankind, and that held by those who are convinced that a progressive hybridization of humans and machines is inevitable, or even desirable (what has been called a cyber-organic species or simply cyborgs), beyond any axiological consideration. This last group, visibly represented by persons like the renowned inventor Raymond Kurzweil [2005], considers that we should develop a pure technology model without ethical restrictions; they base their optimism on a kind of enthusiasm for technology and its benefits. They hold that genetics, nanotechnology and robotics will create a species of unrecognizably high intelligence, memory, durability, comprehension capacity, and so on. Humankind, they think, is at the threshold of a new age of achievements and happiness. However, if the ethical considerations are set apart and machines in our bodies (*nanobots*) can rebuild cells, for example, why could not they be reengineered as weapons? They seem to forget considerations of this and other types, as those of political and economic nature, and the fundamental fact that technology needs massive social acceptance and confidence. It is not enough to convince us that human ingenuity is unlimited and can make possible most of our dreams; it is also necessary to convince us that such developments are desirable. We are, certainly, the most well-informed society in history, but ... are we the wisest?

What can support the optimism of the other group, those who do not accept an uncontrolled development of technology and want to preserve human values and nature as we know them today? Well, they must base their optimism on evidence rather than speculations. Along history humankind has seen a considerable improvement of life conditions and physical progress, in spite of wars and natural catastrophes. Man has been a very successful species in controlling his surroundings and developing a production capacity to meet his needs and make true his dreams. The dire predictions made in the past about the limited capacity for food production in comparison to population growth had vanished thanks to technology. And the same is true in connection with other commodities. In 1798 Malthus published his classical work on his catastrophic predictions about the impossibility of feeding human population due to the fact that food production was growing linearly while human population increases at a geometrical rate. Two hundred years later Malthus predictions are far from being confirmed, although from time to time a new version of Malthusian arguments alerts us about the proximity of a new crisis. Among these Neo-Malthusians we found at the end of the 1960's the Club of Rome [Meadows, 2004]: they feared that the earth was rapidly running out of everything due mainly to the fast population growth. In 1968 Paul Ehrlich, a respected biologist from Stanford University and president of Stanford's Center for Conservation Biology, published *The Population Bomb* [Ehrlich, 1971], in which he posited that sustainability is determined by three basic factors: population, resources availability and technology. The basic argument was this: more people imply more poverty, which in turn implies more people. This book stimulated the movements looking for accomplishment of zero population growth. Some years later appeared the book *The Limits to Growth*, from a group of researchers working at the Massachusetts Institute of Technology, headed by Denis L. Meadows under request of The Club of Rome. They studied five indicators related to economy: population growth, resource consumption, technological development, food production, and pollution. Using a computer model and the best data they could find at the time for these indicators, they concluded that "if the present trends continue unchanged, the limits to grow on this planet will be reached sometime within the next 100 years" [Meadows, 1992]. Nevertheless, they

left open the possibility of altering these growth trends and to establish a condition of ecological and economic stability that can be sustainable far into the future.
Fortunately, none of these apocalyptical visions have come true. In 1980 the economist and expert in administrative sciences Julian L. Simon published a book [*The Ultimate Resource*, 1996] which contained a good deal of arguments intended to prove that population growth is not by itself a menace. His reasoning was on the line of "both, foxes and people like to eat chickens; but while more foxes mean less chickens, more people means more chickens". In other words, the larger the human population that can create and invent, the easier for a society to raise its production and living standards. Simon's central premise was that people are the ultimate resource: "Human beings", he wrote, "are not just more mouths to feed, but are productive and inventive minds that help find creative solutions to man´s problems, thus leaving us better off over the long run". In the average, a person using modern technologies can produce more than he or she consumes. According to Simon, natural resources are getting less scarce, world food supply is improving, world pollution is being controlled, and population growth has long-term benefits. Having opposing visions, Ehrlich and Simon entered in a famous wager in 1980, betting on a mutually agreed-upon measured of resource scarcity over the decade leading up to 1990. Ehrlich chose five commodity metals; Simon bet that their prices would decrease and Ehrlich bet they would increase. Ehrlich ultimately lost the bet, and all five commodities that were selected as the basis for the wager continued to trend downward during the wager period.
The two trends that Simon believed best represented the long-term improvement in the human condition along history due to the technological development, were the increase in life expectancy and the decrease in infant mortality. Those trends, Simon maintained, were the ultimate sign of man´s technology victory over his problems.
Anyhow, the debate between optimists and pessimists is not yet settled, but if we consider that optimism is more an attitude than a vision of the expected then the only way to give sense to the human actions based on our best rational efforts is to keep by principle an optimistic stand, since any alternative could not favor life. As we have seen, if the positive results of the applications of new technologies were balanced against the risks involved, no doubt the first would prevail when used with prudence. That is the challenge of our times.

7. Conclusions

Up to now technology has been an instrument of man to control nature in search of better living conditions. As any living organism, technology has evolved in an almost continuous way by incremental innovations to become, at present times, a very complex system that is developing its own laws and its own government. Then, we have to be cautious not to be controlled by our own creation [Roe-Smith & Marx, 1994].
On the other hand, if the success of a technology is measured by its beneficial effects on human life, then the most successful of all modern technologies are those related to human health; perhaps because these are the most visible results for the majority of the people. However, the climate change, the foreseen energy crisis, as well as biotechnologies, genetics engineering, telecommunications and Internet, together with its implications for human life and values, are forcing us to wake up from the "technological somnambulism" envisioned by Winner [2008], to abandon passivity and take a more active role in orienting and controlling the future technological development. It is too much what is in stake to let the experts or politicians alone make the job of decision taking. And we cannot forget that we

will make our decisions about technology in a world built by technology itself, so we are constrained by what past technology has made of our world; we are not entirely free to choose a course of action. Nevertheless, the sooner we assume a participative role the more effectively we can steer our future and choose the kind of world we wish for our descendants. One thing we can take for granted: technological progress cannot -and should not- be stopped, since it is inherent to human nature. We cannot go back to earlier periods of history, but at the same time we must struggle to have the kind of progress that can provide the greatest benefits for all of us. And following Peter Drucker [2011] we could conclude that: ".... A time of true technological revolution is not a time for exultation. It is not a time for despair either. It is a time for work and for responsibility."

8. Acknowledgements

The authors, members of the Sistema Nacional de Investigadores-México, acknowledge the support if this institution and are also indebted to the Instituto Politécnico Nacional de México for providing the funds for this work through the Project SIP-20110453.

9. References

Arthur, W. B. (2009). *The Nature of Technology. What it is and How it Evolves*, Free Press, ISBN 978-1-4165-4405-0, New York, USA

Churchland, P. S. (2011). *Braintrust: What Neuroscience Tells Us about Morality*, Princeton University Press, ISBN 978-0-691-13703-2, New Jersey, USA

Drucker, P. F. (2011). *Technology, Management, and Society*, pp. 108-119, Harvard Business Review Press, ISBN 978-1-4221-3161-9, Boston, Massachusetts, USA

Dyson, F. (1993). Science in Troubles, The American Scholar, Vol. 62, No. 4, (Autumn 1993), pp. 513-525, ISSN 0003-0937, Washington, D. C., USA

Ehrlich, P. R. (1971). *The Population Bomb*, Buccaneer Books, ISBN 1-56849-587-0, New York, USA

Ferrer, J. J. & Álvarez, J. C. (2003). *Para Fundamentar la Bioética*, Editorial Desclée De Brouwer, ISBN 84-330-1814-0, Bilbao, España

Hauser, M. D. (2006). *Moral Minds. The Nature of Right and Wrong*, Harper Collins, ISBN 978-0-06-078072-2, New York, USA

Ho, M. W. (1998). *Genetic Engineering: Dream or Nightmare?* Continuum Press, ISBN 84-7432-743-1, New York, USA

Kelly, K. (2010). *What Technology Wants*, Penguin Books, ISBN 978-0-670-02215-1, New York, USA

Kurzweil, R. (2005). *The Singularity is Near: When Humans Transcend Biology*, Penguin Books, ISBN 0-670-03384-7, New York, USA

Laín-Entralgo, P. (1994). Técnica, Etica y Amistad Médica, In *Memorias*, II Simposio Internacional "Humanismo y Medicina", pp. 27-36, Fondo de Cultura Económica, ISBN 968-16-4608-8, México

Lightman, A.; Sarewitz, D. & Desser, C. (2003). *Living with the Genie, Essays on Technology and the Human Quest for Human Mastery*, Island Press, ISBN I-55963-419-7, Washington, D. C., USA

Martínez, J. L., editor, (2003). *Dilemas Éticos de la Medicina Actual. Comités de Bioética*, Editorial Desclée de Brouwer, ISBN 84-3301775-6, Universidad Pontificia Comillas, España.

Meadows, D. H.; Meadows, D. L. & Randers, J. (1992). *Beyond the Limits: Confronting Global Collapse, Envisioning a Sustainable Future*, Chelsea Green Publishing Co., ISBN 0-930031-55-5, Vermont, USA

Meadows, D. H.; Randers, J. & Meadows, D. L. (2004). *The Limits to Growth. The 30 Years Update*, Chelsea Green Publishing Co., ISBN 1-931498-51-2, Vermont, USA.

Ortega y Gasset, J. (2005), Obras Completas, Vol. III, Ediciones Taurus, ISBN 978-84-306-0580-4, Madrid, España

Potter, V. R. (1988). *Global Bioethics: Building on the Leopold Legacy*, Michigan State University Press, ISBN 978-0870-13264-3, Michigan, USA

Ridley, M. (2010). *El Optimista Racional*, Ediciones Taurus, ISBN 978-6-0711-0766-4, México.

Roe-Smith, M. & Marx, L., editors, (1994). *Does Technology Drive History?* The MIT Press, ISBN 0-262-69167-1, Cambridge, Massachusetts, USA

Schweber, S. S. (2000). *In the Shadow of the Bomb: Oppenheimer, Bethe, and the Moral Responsibility of Scientist*, Princeton University Press, ISBN 0-691-04989-0, New Jersey, USA

Simon, J. L. (1996). *The Ultimate Resource*, Princeton University Press, ISBN 0-691-04269-1, New Jersey, USA

Winner, L. (2008). *La Ballena y el Reactor. Una Búsqueda de los Límites en la Era de la Alta Tecnología*, 2da. Edición, Editorial Gedisa, ISBN 978-84-7432-280-4, Barcelona, España

5

Public Health Bioethics

Miguel Kottow
Escuela de Salud Pública Universidad de Chile, Chile

1. Introduction

The approach of bioethics to the theory and practice of public health is recent and tentative, leading to a highly controversial field of inquiry, and equally polemic normative proposals. In spite of its enormous academic popularity, bioethics has been criticized and faulted for excessive theoretical zeal, and a penchant for highly specific issues that ignore the problems of health and disease at a more global level. Bioethics frequently indulges in holistic ethical language that appears vacuous and unrealistic, unable to come up with practical suggestions for everyday decision-making.

Applied ethics is concerned with ethical questions and dilemmas arising in social practices; consequently, bioethics encompasses ethical reflection across the whole gamut of biomedical practices including clinical, public health, and research aspects. The bioethical understanding of such a complex social reality as public health requires a working knowledge of the historical development and actual scope of public health, a daunting task that needs to be at least cursorily approached, especially since mapping the agenda of public health will lead to address such disparate disciplines as ethics and axiology –the study of values-, cultural perspectives, sociological, epistemological and general philosophical questions. Defining and refining concepts involves values, thus showing *ab initio* that [bio]ethics is inextricably interwoven in the social practice of public health. An yet, there is no widespread agreement whether the moral aspects of public health should be understood as professional ethics or, rather, as a branch of the recently developing discipline of bioethics.

To introduce the theory and practice of ethics into public health would be extemporaneous if strictly based on traditional views derived from deontology, utilitarianism or virtue ethics, all of them concerned with essential and absolute concepts like Right or Wrong, Good or Evil, and Virtue versus Sin. Aristotele, Kant and Mill are all at the foundations of ethical thought, but the language employed in applied ethics has inevitably changed. Nor is it appropriate or sufficient to develop a code of professional ethics in the hope of dealing with the intricate problems of complex social practices.

During these initial decades and up to the turn of the century, public health and bioethics ignored each other, except for sporadic academic events unimaginatively concerned with the professional ethics of epidemiologist and public health officials: honest research, collegial competition, scientific solidarity and acknowledgment of peers' originality and priority. Publications dealing with specific issues related to public health were gathered into anthologies [Beauchamp & Steinbock, 1999] but such efforts were insufficient to lay the foundations of a new field of inquiry or to offer a systematic and normative approach to the ethics of a complex social practice, prompting a leading figure of public health to lament that "public health cannot develop an ethics until it has achieved clarity about its own identity; technical expertise and methodology are not substitutes for conceptual coherence." [Mann, 1997].

The first generation of publications devoted to the subject of normative ethics in public health, presented a corpus of professional ethics [Fayerweather, Higginson & Beauchamp, 1991] that led to the elaboration of the American Public Health Association Code of Ethics [Kass, 2001]. The main thrust of this effort was to present the ethical implications of public health activities, and to emphasize the need for a normative blueprint to act correctly *in* the practice of its scientific, technical, economic, and political activities. Beyond these normative efforts, it now seems appropriate to apply terms and concepts of bioethics in dealing with the ethics *of* public health, the quest for excellence and the deliberation on rights and duties, autonomy, beneficence and fairness due to all those affected by biomedical practices. Bioethics deliberation on public health activities engrossed in the prevention of disease and the promotion of health, will only be true to its self-set goals if it addresses the needs and desires of all those involved: providers, planners and practitioners, beneficiaries, the common weal and, as some scholars are proposing, the ultimate and perhaps illusionary attainment of global justice.

Public health itself has also come under scrutiny because it takes for granted that its constituent terms are clear and univocal. But that is far from true; indeed, there have been many proposals to change the name of the discipline to social, communitarian, collective, population or even global health, and cogent arguments in favor of each of these denominations are presented. Does 'public' refer to a group, an association, a community? Or does it refer to the actual, or perhaps only the legal, inhabitants of a nation? Should one refer to regional or even global population as the public?

Health is an equally elusive concept, poorly served by the holistic World Health Organization's [WHO] definition -well-being at the biological, psychological and social levels-, which begins by being counterintuitive in its denial of health as the absence of disease, and the neglect of common sense acceptance that people who are not sick should be considered healthy. There are intermediate positions based on well-thought arguments that resist perfunctory dismissal, but have been discussed elsewhere [Caplan, Engelhardt Jr., McCartney, 1981]. Refined diagnostics and molecular biology dictate that latency and predispositions will render relative the idea of absent disease. And, at the other end of the spectrum, the boundaries of what health means are expanded by developing selective and enhancing interventions in a quest for excellence and performance beyond normalcy.

A fairly succinct and traditional definition of public health sees it as "the science and the art of preventing disease, prolonging life and promoting physical health through organized community efforts" [Winslow 1920, cited in Gostin, 2002]. What is the place of art in a discipline that is based on scientific research yielding information for technically efficient interventions? Prolonging life hardly seems a primary goal of public health, it is rather a consequence of well-designed policies and programs carried out in a socioeconomic and ecological favorable environment. And do organized efforts of society mean that citizens take care of themselves in healthcare issues? An even more Spartan definition may ease the way into a better focused and more fruitful discussion: "Public health is what we, as a society, do collectively to assure the conditions for people to be healthy." [Institute of

Medicine, 1988, cited in Gostin, 2002]. Interestingly, ethical emphasis is added by confirming "[S]ociety's obligation to assure the conditions for people's health."[Gostin, 2002].

Some preliminary insight may be gained by briefly reviewing the history of public health and the development of bioethics. But historical perspectives should be approached with caution, for different parts of the world will show unequal levels of public health development. National societies simultaneously harbor a variety of policies and approaches to public health issues, due to differing socioeconomic determinants of health and disease, to contextual and often arbitrary allocation of resources, and to the profound impact of social, health and healthcare inequities and gradients. Especially in less developed countries, traditional public health efforts at controlling infectious diseases will coexist with a high prevalence of non-communicable morbidity, due to class differences where whole segments of populations live in colonial-like poverty while others, few but influential, belong to the exclusive caste of the immensely rich. Disparities in income show a Gini Index of 0.45-0.50 (gross inequity) for Latin American nations compared to around 0.30 (moderate inequity) in developed countries.

2. The development of public health

Plagues, a word rooted in *plāga* meaning divine punishment, were believed to be caused by godly wrath as punishment for human misdeeds; such major catastrophes were to be suffered without eliciting action beyond repentance and prayer. Egyptian theurgy recognized Sekhmet as the goddess of pestilence, easily aroused and requiring careful and devoted appeasement. Hippocratic writings show clear awareness that diseases do not only befall the individual human body, but also may lodge in communities -endemics- or suddenly strike whole populations -epidemics-, this being due to the local peculiarities of "airs, waters, places" as discussed in "An essay on the influence of climate, water supply and situation on health". The Hippocratics classified diseases that were of necessity incurable and mortal *-kat'anánken-*, in contrast to fortuitous disorders amenable to medical ministrations *-katà tykhen-*. In "Epidemics", diseases are dramatically depicted, mostly running a relentless course towards death. As so often in Greek medicine, the physician's concern is limited to recognizing the disease and predicting its outcome, lest he be made responsible for injudiciously interfering with untreatable conditions [Lloyd, 1978].

The awareness of population health and disease was broached more pragmatically by the Romans, who assiduously followed Cicero's dictum *salus populi suprema lex est* -health of the population is supreme law-, where *salus* referred to well-being, but also to salvation and health. Romans' incipient public health measures were directed towards securing water supply, supervising public baths, and building sewerage systems to keep a clean city. Thus, Augustus and his *aediles* appeared to ignore the belief held in antique societies concerning the divine origin of diseases and man's impotence to deviate the course of natural events.

Nevertheless, the Middle Age recurrently mingled magical thinking with faith and the belief that diseases were caused by *fatum* or destiny, that is, divine punishment for moral turpitude, as compared to morbid conditions due to *fortuna* or chance, where medical interventions were indicated. Hygienic measures were for the most part practiced in monasteries, leaving city dwellers unprotected. The great pandemics that ravaged Europe well into the 17th century were described as "visitations that struck from" heavens, which did not abate till the moment it "pleased God", for "vain was the help of man" [Defoe,

1722]. City administrators registered the appearance, dissemination, and final disappearance of these virulent bouts, seeing their main task in isolating the sick and instructing the healthy to emigrate, or at least keep to themselves, and applying measures aimed at preventing contagion even though the actual mechanisms of transmission were unknown. In his much celebrated History of Public Health, [Rosen] (1993) prefers to speak of prophylaxis rather than prevention, for the traditional public health measure in the wake of epidemic outbursts was confined to establishing barriers to isolate the sick and protect the healthy. Prophylaxis resorted to quarantine, sealing infected houses, interning the sick in hospices, leprosy-houses *-lazzaretos-*, pox-houses *-Blaternhäuser-* and wood-houses *-Holzhäuser-*. Daniel Defoe's account of the bubonic plague that ravaged London in 1648, depicts public health officials dictating strict measures of defensive prophylaxis while helplessly observing the course of events. Isolation was so drastic as to be resisted as immoral, for if disease was suspected in one individual, the whole house-hold was locked in, incarcerating all its inhabitants including those not yet afflicted. Fleeing infested cities was another prophylactic measure, mostly reserved for the affluent, often condemned by Reformist Christians who believed that fate, not human decision, would spare the worthy. Other dignitaries of the cloth took the opposite view, urging their parishioners to fulfill their religious duty of escaping to avoid infection and death [Cunnigham & Grell, 2000].

Epidemics were due to external factors, much as Hippocrates had suggested, leading Sydenham to speak of an atmospheric "epidemic constitution", the origin of which were emanations from the earth, the *miasmas*. The atmospheric-miasmatic theory survived up to the 19th century, complemented by the idea of some self-propagating and transmissible particle which Fracastoro in the 16th century considered to be a seed or *seminaria*, as was eventually proven by Pasteur, Koch and the nascent discipline of bacteriology.

This brief account illustrated the intertwinement of public health problems with moral and religious considerations, superseded but never quite eliminated by modernity's reliance on reason and science.

2.1 Political dimensions of public health

Rosen considers the political birth of the nation-state as the most important impulse for the rising awareness of public health challenges that led to disciplined programs of hygiene and the policing of population behavior. After the Peace of Westphalia (1648), empires were replaced by nation-states with clearly demarcated, although often disputed, territorial limits and the political mandate to take care of the inhabitant population. The State required political administration based on policies and revenues, both aspects needing a quantitative evaluation of populations in terms of demographic data and productivity, as well as estimates of available resources. Being, as Rosen quotes, "the art or reasoning by figures upon things relating to government", it is hardly surprising that the term "statistics" should have been coined by Achenwall in 1749 "to designate the descriptive analysis of the political, economic, and social organization of states."

Trade and commerce were the most important activities in European countries during the Renaissance, benefiting society and the state by way of accumulating power. The politics and economics of power known as mercantilism were carried out for the benefit of an authoritarian sovereign; in Germany, the term cameralism aptly described the nation's productive efforts at filling the emperor's coffers. Such an efficient production machinery required the working population to remain healthy and disciplined, inspiring B. Ramazzini to publish the first comprehensive treatise on occupational medicine (1700), and J.P. Frank to present his *System einer vollständigen medicinischen Polizei* (1779), which ran through six editions in 30 years [Carrol, 2002].

As the State took over the governance of its people, it began to record birth and death data, culling demographic statistics of population health and disease conditions, in order to give substance to a new form of politics that came to be known as biopolitics [Foucault 2008, cited in Macey, 2009]. During the 19th century, the triumphs of public health measures based on the theory of *miasma* were superseded by bacteriology and the demonstration that the transmission of infectious diseases was due to contagion by microorganisms. Further demographic and epidemiological developments inaugurated the present era of chronic diseases resistant to curative efforts, leading to intense scientific research, and major changes in public health strategies. Thus, three eras of public health are recognized, presenting epidemiological turns in the wake of demographic and socioeconomic developments:

- Medical police and biopolitics -17th to 19th century-.
- Infectious diseases and the search of a *causa vera* inspiring epidemiological research in the 19th and initial 20th century.
- Degenerative diseases informed by multicausal thinking, extensive epidemiological research, increased awareness of socioeconomic determinants of health and disease and, in due time, the development of a new public health culture.

The purpose of the present text is to follow the bioethical implications of these demographic and epidemiological transitions which are less clearly demarcated in underdeveloped countries, where endemic infections coexist with a mounting prevalence of chronic degenerative conditions.

3. Bioethical issues in public health

Clinical ethics had evolved from the placid and bloodless sort of medical ethics known since Hippocrates, through Percival and up to the first half of the 20th century, when a new era of scientific medicine woke up to a host of quandaries about the right thing to do, facing the requirements of a more sturdy moral discipline that led to the birth of bioethics in the early 1970s. Clinical bioethics became involved in unsettling issues like autonomy and fairness, the elusive concepts of health and disease, care of the disadvantaged and the mentally incompetent, the responsible attitude towards biomedical research subjects, the relevance of biomedical investigations. Academic bioethics flourished, getting so involved with scholarly fine points of theory, that it seemed to lose touch with reality and become irrelevant to the needs and worries of the biomedical practices it was expected to study and influence [Hedgecoe, 2004].

Few scholars resisted the temptation of simply transcribing bioethical principlism to the public health agenda, failing to remember that the so-called Georgetown mantra was itself an adaptation to clinical practice of the Belmont Report (1978/79), issued as a ethical guide for biomedical research with human beings. The Belmont Report and the shortly thereafter presented and highly influential principle-based brand of bioethics addressed the one-to-one, face-to-face doctor/patient and researcher/subject relationship, thus offering scarce enlightenment to the collective and anonymous practices of public health programs [Beauchamp & Childress, 2001].

Ethical problems applied to the many diverse aspects of public health practices, can basically be grouped under five headings. The most pervasive and amply recognized area of conflict occurs in evaluating the common good and its requirements versus individual autonomy. Secondly, the tendency of public authorities to impose policies often clashes with scientific information, or lack of it, about what to do or omit. Thirdly, the eternal dichotomy of *natura/cultura* is reenacted as epidemiology explores biological, especially molecular, predispositions and risk, with diminished concern for sociological factors that influence these dispositions. Fourth, socioeconomic determinants are presented and contrasted with theoretical suggestions of reforms, empowerment, the quest for justice and health equity, at the same time forging public health policies that seek to promote health by influencing freely adopted life-styles. Finally, the impact of globalization and its consequences on human rights approach to public health will be briefly discussed.

3.1 Collective goals and individual autonomy

The crux of public health bioethics may well be the conflict between individuals and society, for public health is always a collective enterprise that needs to be implemented by acting on individuals or requiring their cooperation. Immunization is a typical public health intervention, but it consists of vaccinating individuals. In the era of epidemics, the severity of plagues was assessed by recording the number of deaths occurring per unit of time, based on the idea of society as an aggregate of individual human beings. The strong resurgence of neoliberal politics has given new impulse to the idea of monadic individuals who are assembled rather than interrelated: "particular interventions aim at the health of the public…they should promote health on such a scale that it is visible in aggregate population health figures." (Veveij & Dawson, 2007).

The final aim of public health does not differ from medicine's efforts and goals to prevent and treat disease, and promote health in the individual, the difference rather being that public health addresses the collective factors that influence health and disease, and promotes communal interventions that could not be carried out by individual efforts alone. Recognizing the complex interaction between the common weal and individual autonomy focuses the basic ethical perspective needed to analyze, justify and orientate the moral solvency of public health.

By definition, public health addresses issues that affect society at large, specific communities, or groups. Although helpful interventions are expected to benefit most members, it does not follow that specific individuals will be among the favored, as the well-known "preventive paradox" illustrates: "A preventive measure which brings much benefit to the population offers little to each participating individual,"[Rose, 1985] One of the reasons bioethics needs to be incorporated into public health is to provide rational ethical arguments that should help clarify when public health is justified in imposing policies as compared to situations where individual autonomy is reasonably invoked in opposition to public demands.

Social interests and care of the common weal are habitually understood as responsibilities of the State acting through democratic, and hopefully participative, governmental institutions. A new field of controversy is thus created, because the State may be constitutionally liberal or even libertarian and therefore partial to only minimal intervention in social affairs, or it may harbor a strong social persuasion to provide more expansive welfare tasks. Accordingly, health protection and care can be carried out by governmental institutions, private initiative or a mixture of both, involving a variety of political views and ethical concerns. Throughout history and in different societies, the balance between the collective/individual, and the State/market alternatives has shifted, creating polemics and requiring normative adjustments, as well as ethical reconsiderations.

Even if a public program appears to be widely beneficial, certain individuals may wish to be exempted, preferring to seek the same benefits on their own. For example, massive vaccination may be individually objected on the ground that privately purchased immunization is more convenient. Others might seek exemption because they do not believe in the expected benefits, or fear harmful consequences -allergies, negative reactions of underlying disease, or unpleasant side-effects-.

Believers in public action will argue that the common weal ought to take precedence over individual preferences, and such a position is probably justified provided that: a) it is demonstrably certain that the public will benefit from the intended action; b) the program may be less effective if individual dissent is accepted; c) dissenters have valid arguments that could survive the scrutiny of expert questioning. Therefore, public health measure that are compulsory when disciplined and universal participation is technically necessary to ensure effectiveness, leave little room for individuals opting out. In health promotion activities, on the other hand, where the public is merely being informed and certain conducts are recommended but not enforced, dissenters may freely ignore such campaigns.

It has been recognized that "(given limited resources) monies allocated to public health may come at the expense of monies for treating acute clinical care." This clearly sets out a dichotomy of community versus the individual [Boylan, 2008]. The tension between individuals and society is not only a matter of conflicting personal cooperation or dissent with needs and goals of the common weal, it may also involve resources allocation. The right to receive urgently needed scarce resources will conflict with the public mandate to reasonably ration resources in order to assign them in the best interest of all.

Scholars have defended privileging the endangered individual to the detriment of public benefits. For the sake of rhetoric, "rescue" is limited to life-saving interventions under the assumption that no alternative can trump over preserving life [Quigley & Harris, 2008]. The situation is a special case of the more general dilemma between allocating resources to public health endeavours or to medical therapy, a dilemma that, but for rare exceptions, has been consistently solved in favour of tertiary medical care. In fact, many nations allow insufficiently funded public health to coexist with costly and sophisticated medical services.

In defending rescue medicine, it is postulated that its beneficiaries are identifiable, whereas public interventions are "statistical and non-identifiable" but, if this argument is allowed to prevail, funds would invariably flow to individual treatment, for the common weal pursued by public health is always anonymous. Secondly, it is said that rescue interventions are of immediate or short-term benefit, whereas public prevention measures are effective, if at all, in the distant future. In spite of its numerous critics, discounting the future is a valid argument, but not because future generations are too distant to stimulate protection, but because vast number of actually living human beings are in dire need which cannot be bypassed in favour of the undetermined future. Discounting the future is further justified because expected benefits for as yet unborn generations will also obtain from present environmental policies. Failing to discount the future means planning benefits for future generations at the cost of neglecting contemporaneous needs. Securing resources for the future is only reasonable and justified if presently unmet needs have been covered. Environmental ethics, for example, envisions policies and interventions that will improve natural conditions for living beings in the future, but the actual implementation of such measures will be of present benefit as they reduce rates of deterioration, pollution and exploitation.

3.2 Public domain and private realm

The potential conflict between collective goals and individual rights to non-interference has been presented as two opposing sociological perspectives. Under the influence of Marx and Durkheim the unit of observed action is always society, i.e., the individual as part of, and determined by, social ties. In contrast, the individualistic approach conceived by Pareto and Weber prefers to understand human actions as initiated by singular persons, modulated but not determined by their social circumstances [Van der Maesen & Nijhuis, 2000]. In the first view, economic and social influences inform and permeate each human being, whereas emphasis on the individual entails recognizing free will that is autonomous and called upon to resist coercion from external determination.

The collective/individual dichotomy is closely related to the issue of public domain versus private realm, state-centred political arrangements versus libertarian non-interference, finally debating upon the proper area of concern for healthcare as a public intervention versus an individual, self-responsible enterprise.

Ever since the mid 1800s, public health began collecting statistical data on biological processes such as birth and mortality rates, health conditions, and life-expectancy, leading to political interventions described as "population biopolitics" [Foucault, 2008, cited in Macey, 2009]. The prevention of epidemics, the fluoridation of water supply, the imposition of safety measures, or the regulation of production and distribution of food and drugs are some examples were disciplined cooperation of all citizens is required, avoiding any form of individual non-compliance, lest the public health goals derive in failures and increased risks. Enforcing public health measures considered to be essential may entail impositions and sanctions, coercing individual autonomy to a point that many citizens might resent. From a sociological point of view, the public space has been expanding its field of influence to include and invade the private realm with the purpose of inducing, even regulating, personal conduct. Dissuasive recommendations and legal restrictions are part of the political life of many nations, affecting personal decisions in areas like reproduction, sexuality, disease, and dying. "The distance between civil society and the State increases, whereas the separation between private and public life is disappearing."[Touraine, 1985]

These are more than merely academic debates, for many countries, especially of the Third World, validate strict and mandatory public health policies regarding suicide, euthanasia, the right to reject life-saving medical intervention, abortion, assisted reproduction, availability of contraception, organ donation. Evidence has been presented that under the banner "culture of life", prosperous countries have earmarked political, economic, and public health support to poor populations, by requiring recipient countries to actively combat prostitution, prohibit abortion, or promote abstinence as the primary preventive against HIV infection [Purdy 2008].

In view of such ethical transgressions of public health interventions, it is hardly surprising that individual autonomy defenders should become suspicious and vigilant, leading to unsettled opposition between public health policies and the preferences of civil society's members. The abortion controversy is a prime example of social desires and needs that are opposed by recalcitrant public policies, leading to unsafe clandestine interventions, unwanted children and child abuse, socioeconomic deterioration, and increased suffering of families living in poverty. The pro-life / pro-choice polemic is a clear illustration of an unresolved and ongoing clash between the social vocation of religious and conservative institutions to safeguard a "right to life", and the claim for unhindered reproductive decisions in the private realm.

At the political level, collectivism tends to support a strong, democratic and participatory State, engaged in promoting the common weal in an atmosphere of social justice that is expected to meet the basic needs of all citizens. A strong State is essential in nations where inequities marginalize and disempower important segments of the population who are in need of support to gain access to basic goods: nutrition, healthcare, education and social security. Neoliberalism as well as its libertarian version, reject any intervention beyond the minimal State that protects life, patrimony and national territory, expecting individuals to seize equal opportunities and autonomously shape their lives. Libertarianism presumes all inhabitants of the nation to be citizens, i.e., have their basic rights respected and their national affiliation recognized, enabling them to have unhindered access to the social arrangements that guarantee law and order. Public health is profoundly affected by these divergent views regarding the political, philosophical and bioethical aspects it must consider, as can be illustrated by reviewing the evolution of epidemiology, and changes in its research objectives.

3.3 Epidemiology: Quest for knowledge

Epidemiology has evolved into a scientific inquiry focused on the demographic distribution and causes of disease and health related processes, gathering evidence to inform and sustain public health in its preventive and promotional activities. Influenced by demographic transitions, epidemiology has been modifying its epistemological perspectives and research methods. Different denominations and taxonomies have been proposed, one of the most illustrative being presented by Susser & Susser [1996], who characterize the evolution of epidemiology in four eras, each developing its own paradigm:

EPIDEMIOLOGICAL FOCUS	CONCEPTUAL MODEL
Sanitary statistics	Miasma
Infectious diseases	Germ theory
Chronic diseases	Black box
Eco-epidemiology	Chinese boxes

As previously mentioned, political engagement in hygiene and sanitation based on the miasma theory served to discipline and police the population in the early times of modernity. In the 19th century public health was mainly concerned with infectious diseases, as biomedical research was aiming to find the *causa vera* of diseases, and epidemiology refined its observations on the ways infections were transmitted. Pasteur's bacteriological research and Koch's postulates suggested that infectious diseases were due to identifiable microorganisms, and inspired the search for a specific therapeutic agent, the magic bullet pursued by P. Ehrlich.

These efforts influenced a major demographic and epidemiological transition as the disease pattern shifted from infectious diseases to non-communicable, degenerative and chronic conditions. The monocausal approach to the now prevalent diseases was hopelessly inadequate as it became apparent that many socioeconomic and environmental factors were involved, a fact that was common knowledge but had not been systematically studied. Multicausality was first thought to be structured in an orderly cause-effect sequence but, as the complex relationship of necessary, sufficient and confounding factors was recognized, epidemiology submerged causal interactions into a black box. Scientists were forced to modify their rigorous cause-effect language, and turn to statistical estimates of probability dealing with as yet poorly identified external circumstances and hosts of conditions that triggered disease processes.

The black box metaphor refers to the awareness that health and disease are complex processes of multicausal origin rooted in biology, environmental and socioeconomic contexts, psychological and behavioural processes. Empirical evidence as to the influence of social and economic factors has been so widely accepted as to constitute an array of determinants firmly anchored in reality and resistant to change. New metaphors -networks, Chinese boxes, complex systems-, and denominations like 'eco-epidemiology' have been proposed in order to explain multilayered influences and intricate interactions. The natural and social environmental factors became recognized as strongly pathogenic, and the ideas of eco-epidemiology were introduced and filled with ominous descriptions -unassailable social determinants, global climate changes, irreversible decay of nature-, thus unwittingly supporting a conservative ideology that accepted the *status quo* and discouraged major remedies. The complexities of underdetermination and uncertainty deprived epidemiology of precise and convincing suggestions for preventing diseases and promoting robust healthcare measures, thus denying public health the ethical justification to recruit resources and transform uncertain knowledge into interventions that often become arbitrarily compulsory.

An unedited turnabout occurred as epidemiology became engrossed in studying risk factors and shifting emphasis from external determinants to individual predisposition and exposure. Emphasis was deflected from seeking cause-effect relations to identifying factors of health risk, giving rise to what is now called "risk factor epidemiology" that operates with a penchant for refined probability statistics [Susser, 1998]. Risk is the probability of suffering a negative or deleterious effect and, when uncertainty prevails, there is a tendency to collapse probability into possibility, which means that an event may occur but we have no clue as to the likelihood of it actual occurring. Socioeconomic and environmental risk factors are external to individuals and resistant to modification, as insinuated by naming them determinants rather than conditions. Consequently, risk factors were internalized, research now turning to investigate individual predispositions to deleterious external circumstances. Public health is frustratingly helpless beyond confirming that the poor are especially vulnerable to disease and less able to take care of their health as long as profound socioeconomic changes remain absent. Major changes in the social structure and the distribution of resources are formidable challenges, depending on governmental power and resolution to seek social justice and healthcare equity.

Epidemiological research has come to be considered the irreplaceable scientific basis of public health activities. The bioethics of biomedical research is becoming a major area of deliberation, facing problems that also involve epidemiology: informed consent of individuals and communities, relevance of research projects, private versus public funding, sustainable risks, benefits for research subjects and host communities, and a number of other issues that require ongoing attention. Some of them are briefly mentioned throughout this text, but a few remarks on two salient controversies seem in order: evidence-based epidemiological research, and offshoring.

Evidence-based clinical research has yet to find its place in medical practice and healthcare policies. Hailed as the indispensable foundation of medical knowledge, it has found supporters but also many critics, especially amongst practitioners who lament that experience, contingencies, ethical considerations and patient participation are underrated as decision-making criteria in this scientific approach to treating and caring for the sick. Nevertheless, there is fair agreement that hard evidence is necessary to plan allocation of scarce resources and to set priorities in healthcare programs when legitimate demands exceed availabilities, in which case decisions to ration must rest on well sustained knowledge about efficacy –cost/benefit ratio-, and effectiveness –problem-solving capacity-. Rationing is a complex issue when resources are insufficient to cover essential medical needs, for privileging certain areas will leave others to the dangers of neglect and deterioration.

Evidence-based epidemiology is an elusive goal, since population health is based on complex interactions of many variables and determinants which are practically impossible to dissect for experimental purposes. The quest for probable cause-effect links, in clinical research often focused on dose-response relationships, isolating variables and employing RCT (Randomized Control Trials), is usually insufficient in determining collective disease mechanisms, because statistical probability needs to be supported by plausibility –non randomized observations- and, most important, by adequacy –demonstration that intervention is being effective- [Victora, Habicht & Bryce, 2004]. These technicalities boil down to the fact that linear cause-effect answers rarely satisfy the complexities of public health problems.

Epidemiological research has responded in two ways to these quandaries: First, by accepting external socioeconomic and environmental conditions as given determinants, thus shifting risk factors to the individual where predispositions and disease facilitating behaviour yield information that may be employed in preventive medicine by modifying individual response to rigid external factors. As previously noted, risk factor epidemiology centred on individuals tends to reduce State protection, induce self-care and reinforce the tendency to blame the victim. Secondly, by applying scientific methods in such a rigorous way that reliable internal validity is secured. But, as internal validity increases, results loose external validity, that is, in order to isolate the explored variable, study conditions have been artificially purified in such a way that they differ from real-life conditions to the point of making it implausible to extrapolate results from bench to bedside [Rothman, 1991].

A related problem is offshoring, an inelegant euphemism representing the rapidly increasing tendency of sponsors to carry out research in poor countries, where costs are reduced, ethics standards may be less stringent, and recruiting subjects appears less problematic [Petryna, 2007]. These research protocols, very often carried out by professional research institutions (CRO=Contract Research Organizations), do not heed local needs in their quest for results that are marketable in the original sponsor countries, thus reinforcing the 90:10 divide and the further neglect of the healthcare needs of poor populations.

In view of these new scenarios, a novel form of preventive medicine was developed: accepting that external risk factors were resistant to change, epidemiologic research concentrated on finding out why some individuals and social groups are more susceptible to deleterious circumstances than others. Procedures were developed to identify those at risk, and diagnostic probes refined to map personal vulnerabilities and detect predispositions, focusing on preclinical conditions and early disease manifestations. Molecular biology came to the aid of exploring the biological constitution and genetic flaws of singular human bodies, to the point where rarely anyone manages to emerge with a clean, albeit provisional, health certificate.

3.4 The "new public health"

Post-World War II most European countries became social and well-fare States, though 50 years later financial limitations forced reductive policies, restricted coverage, and increased co-payments for medical services. The undisputed hegemony of neoliberal politics has been wary of too much State intervention, preferring to promote market centred *laissez faire* policies that clip the wings of many public health initiatives. A "new public health" was born, with a neoliberal vocation to shift public health involvement "from the state to members of the public themselves" [Petersen & Lupton, 2000]. This major change in public health philosophy and strategy was strongly supported by the newly developed risk factor epidemiology. The individual at risk is called upon to embark in self-care instead of claiming State protection, every citizen being responsible for a health promoting life-style and advised to seek medical assistance by his own means. As social protection pales, private enterprise flourishes in all areas of medicine and healthcare, thus inevitably exacerbating the inequalities of access and coverage in medical matters [Pearce, 1996].

The marketing of healthcare has influenced biomedical research, which is to an increasing extent dominated by the pharmaceutical industry catering to the needs and desires of the well-off, developing and promoting enhancement medicine, and neglecting research of major and pressing public health problems such as malaria, dengue, and other endemic diseases that ravage poor populations. The term "neglected diseases" was introduced to illustrate the deficiencies of global public health, a term that covered such chilling data as the daily death of 16.000 children from hunger-related causes (Illies, 2008], or of half a million women dying during pregnancy and in childbirth for lack of simple preventive measures [Purdy, 2004].

Medicalization and lucrative enticements for marketing preventive and therapeutic medical interventions have severely increased inequities in healthcare, aggravated by massive brain drain of healthcare professionals. The exorbitant rise of medical care costs are stranding marginal populations, in addition to stimulating medical tourism that entices affluent patients to seek medical care in less developed nations.

Petersen and Lupton [2000] reach the harsh conclusion that "[W]hile new public health authorities and agencies continue to adopt overtly coercive strategies such as quarantine, isolation and enforced medical treatment when they seem required and most justified..., they are equally, if not more, reliant upon the use of strategies that position citizens as acting of their own free will and in their own interests to protect their own health." Public health bioethics must face these accusations and unveil such strategies as are, if not always coercive, steeped in manipulative intents that are ethically suspect and often harmful to individuals and whole populations.

The general trend is to reduce State responsibility in public health matters. Even though recognizing social and economic determinants of health and disease conditions, epidemiological emphasis and new public health proponents are accepting external risk factors as circumstances that individuals have to cope with by actively mitigating their predisposition to be affected by these deleterious circumstances. Adherence to preventive actions and early diagnostic explorations, pre-clinical medication, changes in diet, behaviour and life-style are the bulwarks of responsible self-care. Medicalizing public health increases the vulnerability of citizens with scarce resources, who no longer can find refuge in comprehensive State protection that is either reduced or denied.

3.4.1 The human rights approach to healthcare

From a more global perspective, it appears that different public health paradigms co-exist with changing emphasis throughout time and, to a major degree, in dependence of socioeconomic and cultural diversity. Hygiene, sanitation infrastructure and public health policies mirror the civilization of their time and are strongly determined by the values and beliefs of their social environment [Sigerist, 1960, cited in Mechanic, 1978]. The multicultural trend of modern times, and the coexistence of extreme socioeconomic disparities within societies and across nations, provide strong evidence that public health paradigms overlap and are enmeshed in a permanent turmoil of vested interests, ideological and political motivations, as well as powerful economic influences.

In the second half of the 20th century, Western democracies in Europe expanded social services under the concept of welfare State, including free, universal and comprehensive medical care. For a variety of reasons -massive illegal immigration, lack of resources and personnel, increased costs-, coverage became progressively restricted, although certain basic functions of public health have remained uncontested: immunization, massive screening programs, essential life-saving but extremely expensive interventions and medications like antiretroviral therapy. Although breached in practice, the idea of governmental responsibilities in public health and medical care, especially for the poor and economically feeble population, has remained a valid social and political goal, mainly nurtured by respect for human rights and recognition of a basic right to health [care].

Whether public health [bio]ethics can be adequately and sufficiently grounded in human rights is a matter of ongoing controversy, ranging from the belief that the human rights approach is at the ethical basis of public health, to the objection that rights-talk is too weakly binding to achieve practical results and political commitment, and should be replaced with duty-talk demanding the provision of certain basic public services [Mann, 1997; O'Neill, 1998].

The human rights approach has been counterproductive [Gostin, 2002], because it is unfocused and excessively political "by espousing controversial issues of economic redistribution and social restructuring" [Hessler, 2008]. In fact, international human law has failed to commit national states to binding and enforceable norms; as for the international community, it has been unable to actually inspire political action and social reform, as tragically illustrated by the fact that over 60 years after UNESCO's Universal Declaration of Human Rights one third of the global population suffers from starvation or severe malnutrition, and no less than 3.000.000 children die every year from preventable diseases

[Illies, 2008]. A number of scholars believe that more robust philosophical accounts of human rights are required, stressing that a purely utilitarian approach is too narrow to anchor public health ethics in human rights, especially if moral deliberation is neglected because excessive trust is placed in legal documents.

Acknowledging that "[B]ioethics has gone global", Arras and Fenton support Mann's original idea that bioethics ought to be seen as fundamentally related to the public issue of rights to healthcare, but their analysis leads to some discouraging conclusions: "a right to healthcare goods is incompatible with the unfortunate likelihood that it will not be honored for the majority of the world's poor for many years to come." Therefore, "the lingua franca of human rights, while important and helpful in many ways, is not a sufficient methodological tool for a globalized bioethics." To be effectively action-guiding, human rights need to be embedded in social institutions which in turn are context-bound in their problem-solving capacities. Nations with sparse public health resources will be unable to meet the actual needs and claims that are based on human rights doctrine, leading to the conclusion that "institutional human rights are not, strictly speaking, unmodified *human* rights. They will, rather bear much more resemblance to *political* rights" [Arras & Fenton, 2009]. *Realpolitik* trumps over ethics, leaving global proposals based on human rights to dry out as empty concepts.

3.4.2 Globalization and human rights

Economic expansion and political globalization including the undisputed hegemony of capitalism ever since the collapse of the Soviet Union and East European socialism, has created what N. Fraser has called a postwestphalian macro-political world order [Fraser, 2009]. Transnational business associations in the wake of tendencies to globalize economic strategies and political systems, have had profound impact on many aspects of health, disease and medical care around the world. Globalization has also allowed the powerful to exercise pressure on smaller nations, instigating them to accept the rules of macroeconomy, with their consequences and side-effects.

Public health has suffered from insufficient financial support and a trend towards further reduction of national resources as a consequence of globalizing market policies, as well as the diversion of healthcare monies to insufficiently substantiated promotional campaigns, and to the expansion of extensive anti-bioterrorism strategies. It is well known but rarely publicized, that international banking policies have provided loans to developing countries under the condition that State intervention be reduced, allowing private enterprise to flourish in the market for medical and other social services [Almeida, 2002].

Frequent concern has been voiced about the trend towards privatization and the enormous influence of big medical business, including the pharmaceutical industry, genetic research and its applications, which have marginalized public health efforts at the same as they encourage ideological discourses in favour of global bioethics and global justice.

Global justice, global [bio]ethics, international health equity and similar wide-ranging ethical proposals include acknowledging and fulfilling obligations to the poor, and considerations about distant ethics. These ideas are nurtured by well-known basic facts: socioeconomic determinants of injustice and health inequalities, responsibilities arising from historical political processes -colonialism-, and present economic strategies such as concentration of financial power, monopolistic practices of drug companies and transgenic food producers, big-stick politics in pollution and exploitation of natural resources. And yet, in the wake of powerful and unrelenting economic processes, thinking in terms of global ethics remains an inconsequential academic exercise.The impact of these determinants and macroeconomic policies has been shown to have a nefarious influence on the health condition of the world population, creating inequalities that go hand in hand with increasing social and economic disparities. Wealth and health develop together, as do disease and poverty. Although it remains controversial whether poor health is a major cause of poverty or, to the contrary, lack of essential goods leads to sparse healthcare and precarious disease prevention, it is obvious that a vicious circle ensues between poverty, endemic diseases, lack of resources for medical care and public health programs. International agencies and a number of scholars interested in applied ethics have stressed the urgency of developing acutely needed palliative, remedial and redistributive policies.

An early, general and underdetermined suggestion by the WHO posits that "health inequalities count as inequities when they are *avoidable, unnecessary, and unfair*". Such a candid statement may serve as food for thought, but it will hardly fuel effective strategies to reduce inequities and improve levels of public healthcare: as socioeconomic inequality increases throughout the world, the gradient of health inequality becomes steeper. Does this well documented and often lamented state of affairs generate a transnational obligation to reduce or resolve inequalities or, at least, take steps to avoid that inequity occur, persist and even increase [Singer, 2004; Pogge, 2005]?

Some influential ethical doctrines like Rawls' justice as fairness are meant to apply within national boundaries or, as Nagel puts it, to citizens who "stand in the explicit relation to each other that is characterized by a state". This "statist" perspective is contrasted to a "cosmopolitan" view committed to the belief that justice ought to be a global aspiration, requiring "adequate primary healthcare and basic education [as] preconditions for living a good human life" [Daniels, 2006].

Claiming that many contemporary problems occurring at an international scale render a statist attitude obsolete, globalism envisions "transnationalising the public sphere", in order to foster "new transnational public powers, that possess the administrative capacity to solve transnational problems" [Fraser, 2009]. Public health, which might continue to qualify as a national issue to be approached in a statist fashion is, nevertheless, extremely sensitive to international influences. Control of infectious diseases, for example, is considered to require "comprehensive global efforts" that transcend national prevention programs [Battin et al. 2008]. On the other hand, the 90:10 divide that shows most biomedical research resources to be assigned to the study of health problems affecting the wealthy, is a palpable and depressing illustration how transnational actions deepen inequities by being oblivious to the health needs of the have-not.

In an effort to salvage the cosmopolitan view that international health inequalities ought to be addressed in transnational efforts, Daniels [2008] suggests a minimalist commitment to discourage policies that harm poor nations -brain-draining, aggressive property rights and patent-mongering that limit access to drugs-. In addition, he hopes for the development of a "more promising [relational justice] approach", that will require fair amounts of philosophical groundwork facing vested interest and political divisiveness. Even such well meant top-down approaches remain in the academic realm, for they lack the urgency of those in dire need that require bottom-up practical solutions.

Much writing about universal healthcare rights appears as wishful thinking in the wake of unfulfilled promises of international cooperation and sustained foreign aid commitments [Gordon, 2008]. At a more specific level, offshoring research projects has failed to provide significant post-research benefits to host populations as persistently solicited by the Declaration of Helsinki (Paragraph 17). Furthermore, the Declaration's Paragraph 33 - sharing of post-investigational benefits-, apart from having been watered down in the 2008 version, is regularly honored in the breach, ignored and even vociferously downplayed.

Arguments on global issues are self-interested and myopic, for most nations will agree that a pandemic threatening rich and poor needs to be prevented by collaborative actions. Wealthy nations are willing to engage in military actions in foreign countries, purportedly in defense of global democracy and basic first generation human rights, but will not be equally enthusiastic to participate in supporting improved healthcare and public health programs that honor a right to basic needs including primary healthcare.

Globalization has had additional side effects with epidemiological consequences. Massive migrations have increased the number of displaced and marginalized people who suffer from chronic infectious diseases without having access to proper medical care [Dwyer, 2004]. Migrants who live in camps and are in permanent danger of being evicted or deported, have hardly any prospects of acquiring citizen status, a prerequisite to effective claims of even the most basic human rights. Illegal immigrations bring with them diseases unknown in the host countries, causing hard to manage emergent and resurgent infectious conditions.

A little attended consequence of globalization is brain-drain of healthcare professionals. Trained in a poor country, nurses and doctors are tempted to take jobs in well paid developed nations, leaving their home-population under-staffed and unable to provide basic medical services. Professional migration is stimulated by richer nations that show no qualms in profiting from the educational efforts of poor countries, thus contributing to inequities in healthcare and disregarding their official utterances in favor of global social justice [Dwyer, 2007; Daniels, 2008].

Travel facilities have enhanced tourism and created a new side-line for those seeking medical services abroad. Rising costs are motivating people to explore healthcare facilities in less developed countries, creating an increasing flow of medical tourists, who are attended by qualified professionals and received in luxurious clinics set up in Third World countries that divert resources and man-power from their local public healthcare in order to serve the demands of the traveling patient, making huge profits that remain in the private realm. Local personnel, qualified professionals and resources are sequestered to serve in private facilities, thereby draining the already meager healthcare available to the non-paying indigenous population.

4. The strategies of public health

Public health policies and healthcare programs are mainly inspired by the values of four strategic guide-lines: responsibility, prevention, precaution, and protection, each approach inspired by a different perspective. Although traditionally evaluated in technical terms, there is a growing interest and need to study the ethical justifications and possible limitations of policies that have considerable impact on the well-being of communities and the life of its members, and submit them to public accountability.

FOUR STRATEGIES OF PUBLIC HEALTH INTERVENTIONS	
Strategic concept	**Main theme**
Responsability	causality
Prevention	efficacy
Precaution	opportunity
Protection	empowerment

4.1 Responsibility

Responsibility is the ethical requirement to justify acts, actions or omissions; it differs from accountability in that it goes beyond merely giving account, actually making amends for having caused negative consequences. Accountability is a substantial part of responsibility focused on evaluating resources employed, programs fulfilled and errors committed. The ethical dimensions of responsibility are interwoven with public health in many ways. Search for causes of disease or of failing health is a responsible way of understanding processes, but it also has served to assign blame to the purported causal agent. Responsibility is intrinsic to public health activities performed with serious commitment to efficacy and excellence, and expected to meet the needs of those in distress. From the vantage point of public health, responsibility may be assigned to actions or omissions that cause or facilitate diseases, as well as for instituting preventive healthcare measures, or failing to do so. Thus, public health, being in charge of hygiene and public sanitation, is responsible for its effective procurement, but must also account for and repair failures or undesirable effects [Weed & McKeown, 2003].

When an epidemic is announced, public health institutions are responsible for taking timely and technically appropriate measures to protect the population at risk, by designing and carrying out necessary immunization programs and defence strategies. This responsibility for action is compounded with the obligation to ensure that the measures undertaken are proven to be the best in existence. Failing to intervene, or spending public resources on deficient techniques or polemic goals are examples of responsibilities that must be faced in form of explanation and eventual repair.

Public health responsibilities include socially relevant epidemiological research, and commitment to gain and apply pertinent knowledge to the benefit of society [Weed & McKeown, 2003]. Implicit in this agenda is the much discussed notion that public health ought to engage in active advocacy by shaping activities and setting goals for the sake of the common weal [Krieger, 1999]. These seemingly obvious ethical requirements need to be stressed in view of unfortunate episodes of abuse - eugenic programs, unethical research in Tuskegee Valley and Willowbrook, an ill-advised pandemic alert in 2009-.

As anticipated, the new approach to public health problems has shifted responsibilities by developing the credo of individual self-responsibility in preventing disease and engaging in safe conducts and health promoting life-styles. Reductions of the social element in public health increases healthcare inequities within societies and across nations, as self-care is being negotiated in the medical market rather than in the weakened realm of social security. Scholars reflecting on the reality of less developed countries have voiced their concern that political and economic forces urging individual self-responsibility in healthcare have the intended effect of blunting governmental responsibilities and diluting resources of public health budgets. Implicit in this restructuring is a complex and consequential shift from moral responsibility to economic and legal liabilities, creating litigious situations that consume human efforts and material resources in an infertile endeavour that worsens the reality and options of the underprivileged.

4.2 Prevention

Effective prevention obtains when risks are well defined and can be reduced or eliminated by methods proven to be efficient and sustainable, that is, finding a reasonable and acceptable balance between risk aversion, and negative effects (including costs). Ethical aspects require preventive actions to be indiscriminately available to all those in need of them. From being the defining goal of public health, prevention has been redirected into what came to be known as "Preventive Medicine", referred to "those activities that are in direct responsibility of the individual in the prevention of diseases and the protection of health [Smillie, 1947 as cited in Arouca, 2003]. Preventive medicine advocates have explicitly stressed that preventing disease "should be performed by the medical profession and not through any form of State Medicine" [Fishbein, 1947 as cited in Arouca, 2003]. Thus, much of prevention is deflected from public health policies and incorporated into clinical medicine, therefore addressing individuals rather than populations.

Public health traditionally engages in primary prevention targeted at avoidance of disease. Prevention becomes secondary and tertiary as it mingles with diagnosis and therapy, encouraging self-care and physicians' commitment to pursue disease prevention as part of their clinical practice. The medicalization of prevention leads to periodic and extensive diagnostic explorations in search of predisposing traits of incipient disorders, often resorting to routine prophylactic medication of the healthy. Recently, the term "quaternary prevention" is being employed to sift medical interventions through an ethics filter, and avoid the ill-effects of overmedication. Besides the prevention of iatrogenic effects, some authors suggest that rehabilitation and restoration of function should be the aim of quaternary prevention [Starfield et al, 2008]. The reassignment of many, though not all, preventive measures to prophylactic individual exploration and medication is symptomatic of a major shift from public *health* to clinical *disease*, causing the brunt of prevention to be absorbed by private healthcare organizations and practitioners.

Preventive actions are meant to avert risks and threats to the health of populations. Such actions are required to be effective, avoid unjustifiable and unnecessary interference with the private life of citizens, and target prevalent health problems rather than solely concentrating on individual high relative risk factors. Population-based prevention bases action on collective rather than individual risks. When preventive medicine is carried out as a clinical activity, the destitute in countries with limited resources will rarely get the benefit of preventive measures that have ceased to be governmental responsibility and been taken over by private institutions and healthcare professionals.

4.3 Precaution

A precautionary ethical principle was enounced in the early 1980s as a form of reconciling public acceptance of industrial activities, innovative products, and prevalent technical and extractive processes with their environmental and social impact [Godard, 2001]. Precaution is a decision-rule to be considered in the absence of scientific certitudes about potential consequences of risky situations and processes [Kriebel & Tickner, 2001]. When harmful or irreversible risks to population health actually appear or are strongly suspected, effective and proportionate measures should not be postponed on grounds that scientific and technical knowledge is deemed uncertain or absent. Precaution mandates that whenever harmful risks are suspected but insufficiently defined, action should not be delayed, either to curtail existing situations and activities -post-damage formulation-, or to oppose, eventually postpone, suspicious innovative propositions requiring "safeguarding against serious and, particularly irreversible damage" [COMEST, 2005]. The broad essence of the "precautionary principle is that an action should not be taken when there is scientific uncertainty about its potential impact" [Goldstein, 2001], but critics have rejected such a prematurely sweeping approach because it would inhibit scientific progress and discourage technical innovations [Harris, 2007].

In a climate of uncertainty, precaution means negotiating risks and benefits between proponents of an activity that is under suspicion of being deleterious, and public opinion soliciting regulatory measures aimed at avoiding possible ill-effects. Inasmuch as it is a negotiation in uncertainty, the outcome will often depend on the rhetoric and political force of contending parties. In environmental issues, where little understood variables are the rule and precautionary attitudes are frequently invoked, vested interests will often prevail over civil society's reticence and public health's arguments. Precaution has proven a weak instrument in the hands of social forces unable to curtail the introduction of genetically modified crops and food, technologic sophistications that unleash global warming, or practices that pollute the environment and deplete natural resources.

When judicial conflicts ensue and resort to precautionary arguments, court decisions become unpredictable, for judges may have very different appraisals of risks and uncertainty. The suggested response is to reduce uncertainties, but as knowledge increases precaution should be superseded by well grounded prevention based on precise quantitative risk assessment.

Simplified views on the precautionary principle neglect two important elements: a) Precautionary assessment should involve civil society in order to broaden evaluative criteria; b) Precautionary strategies and the need for robust institutional surveillance require unbiased and uninfluenced politics in order to dictate fair and reasonable regulations and laws.

To apply the precautionary principle with sufficient force to oppose particular interests and devious influence requires control mechanisms capable of collecting and evaluating hard data, advancing a decision-making process based on all eventually available information, and recognizing the major social problems involved [Callon, Lascoumes & Barthe, 2001]. Equally important is the surveillance of public health decisions taken in uncertainty, in order to detect any unwanted effects due to changes in policies inspired by precautionary arguments [Goldstein, 2001].

Excessive precaution and protracted inactivity, it is argued, may stifle progress, just as hasty dismissal of precautionary measures may precipitate disaster, thus warning that precaution is a flexible ethical stance, easily influenced by powerful vested interests, and susceptible to erroneous appraisals. The precautionary principle should also be recursively directed at itself, avoiding its overuse when evidence is clear, certain, and sufficient to inform decisions. Equally, precaution will be inappropriately applied when "there is no reasonable evidence to suspect a risk to public health." [Kriebel & Tickner, 2001].

The 2008 pandemic panic was unleashed by major uncertainties as to the spreading potential of H1N1 virus, and the severity of the infection. WHO was deceitfully misinformed by experts committed to conflicting interests, health officials being erroneously led to recommend massive precautionary measures that depleted public health resources and resulted in huge profits for vaccine producing companies. Pharmaceutical products introduced in the market under the safeguard of precaution have caused severe, even lethal harm, requiring these drugs to be recalled, the thalidomide affair being one of the most dramatic instances: about 25000 children born with atrophic or absent limbs due to a new anti-anxiety drug prescribed to pregnant women. Considering the political weakness of public health institutions and the poor record of precautionary arguments in controlling environmental problems, it seems risky and unreliably to put too much stake on this ethical principle [Marchant, 2003].

In sum, the reliability of the precautionary principle depends on the honesty, good will and ethical solvency of all involved, in the hope that they will be loyal to the maxim of protecting the common weal, and avoid the perils of unknown but potentially deleterious or unwanted effects, as well as the temptations of quick profits obtained without sufficient safeguards.

4.4 Protection

Weary of State intervention, liberal and libertarian political nevertheless agree that even the most minimal State must preserve a solid protective policy towards its citizens and the national territory [Hobbes, 1978; Nozick, 1974]. In addition, the State is responsible for organizing undertakings that will reduce the impact of catastrophic natural events, and defend the population against massive threats –epidemics, scarcity of essential goods, pollution, environmental disasters -.

Protection is needed by those unable to obtain the basic goods required to survive and develop the capabilities that will empower them to plan a meaningful and socially integrated life [Sen, 1995]. The duty to provide essential goods needed for survival are considered to be primary, that is, they are to be served even if no correlative rights are claimed. Although socially recognized rights ought to be secured by correlative obligations, history shows that rights-language is too weak to ensure fulfilment, suggesting that it is more effective to directly demand the execution of essential and uncontroversial obligations. Those in power are under the moral obligation of protecting the weak, the destitute, the damaged and the vulnerable, insofar as they cannot fend for themselves [O'Neill, 1998]. Setting obligations is the correlate of respecting rights, with the advantage that it is a more binding and transparent presentation of what is morally due to human beings. Briefly, the obligation to protect the weak and defenceless can be directly appealed to without the need to proclaim the correlative basic rights, suggesting that talk about a right to health should be replaced with a governmental obligation to provide sanitary and medical protection to the population, at the very least covering the basic needs of the destitute.

In public health, social protection is the counterpart of self-care, invoked by those who admit that healthcare needs ought to be provided to the insolvent, marginalized and otherwise unable to access essential goods and services. Most Latin American Constitutions explicitly concede a right to health, to healthcare or to health protection, to be satisfied through environmental and public health policies, and medical-care services. More broadly, populations are to be protected by reducing the ill-effects of social and economic determinants causing inequities and extreme poor/rich divides, in other words, by aiming to lower the Gini index that measures income disparities, in order to reduce their impact on health inequities. Protection is at the base of a right to healthcare, preferably formulated as the State's obligation to provide indispensable but individually unattainable primary goods

and basic services. The final goal of social ethics will always go beyond the elimination of life-threatening inequities, but hoping for the utopia of attaining global fairness will not feed, heal and educate the poor, who are in dire need of protection.
In a world where the privileged and the economically solvent are minority, States must honour the obligation to provide the basic needs human beings require to survive and function. Duties "are never generated in a vacuum: the idea of needs, and of entitlements based upon needs, always enters in to inform us why the duty is a duty, and why it matters"- [Nussbaum, 2006]. Basic needs are also expressed as lack of the basic capabilities required to survive and project a meaningful life as an integrated member of society. [Sen, 2000]. It is a matter of social justice that the disempowered be protected and assisted by social institutions that specifically address the unattended basic needs of the deprived. Consequently, the essential medical needs of the disempowered become a primary target of social healthcare arrangements, this being another way of calling upon public health to provide basic medical services to the needy who are unable to take care of themselves: "Protection from injury in the face of...ubiquitous and foreseeable vulnerabilities of the human condition is in large measure the task of justice." [O'Neill, 1998]

5. Some special issues

5.1 Infectious diseases

An introductory chapter on public health bioethics can hardly cover all pertinent subjects, so in this fourth part, a few topics have been selected in view of their actuality and importance. Infectious diseases have historically always been in the limelight of public health. New challenges require a reappraisal of well-established ethical norms now facing unprecedented debates and issues that cut across a wide-ranging agenda of public health problems including poverty, global justice, research strategies, public policies, individual responsibility. In recent decades, the emergence and resurgence of treatment resistant infections in affluent societies are again attracting the attention and preoccupation of health officials. Epidemiology is confronted with new and drug-resistant infectious agents, as well as unexpected forms of transmission, to the point where some experts are speaking of a new health transition triggered by the association of infectious and non-communicable diseases [Beaglehole & Bonita, 1997].
Bioethics seems to have neglected a thorough debate on the ethics related to infectious diseases, preferring to delve in the more eye-catching problems of abortion, euthanasia, molecular biology and, more recently, neuroethics and nanoethics [Selgelid, 2005]. The HIV/AIDS scourge, the increasing incidence of drug-resistant tuberculosis, and the unabated force of endemic diseases such as malaria and dengue, are bringing to light a complex array of ethical problems related to their unpredictable epidemiological behaviour.
Bioethics has been criticized for preferably delving in topics related to sophisticated scientific and technological developments, to the detriment of significant problems posed by infections. In their quest for novelty and originality, scholars have failed to take note that industrial development and technological impacts on the environment are changing the landscape of diseases caused by microorganisms and transmitted by unexpectedly aggressive vectors -urbanized rodents, insecticide-resistant arthropods, historically harmless bacteria turned virulent-.

The tension between the communitarian goals of public health and individual autonomy shows peculiarities of its own in the area of infections, considering that each person may become a victim and a vector of infectious diseases. Individuals are called upon to cooperate and behave in a disciplined fashion, as is habitual in most public health policies. As a potential source of contagion, individuals have to protect themselves, as well as behave in such a way as not to infect others nor facilitate the spread of an epidemic bout [Battin et al, 2008]. The responsibility of combating modern infections is shared between public health efforts and individual discipline, not forgetting that clinical medicine must account for the way it employs antibiotics, and is expected to avoid the proliferation of resistant microorganisms, without neglecting fair and cost-conscious prescriptions.

The ethics of public health in dealing with infectious diseases must rely on some kind of regulations and impositions. A drug-resistant TBC infection may require isolation of affected patients, just as VIH (+) individuals are mandated to inform their condition to sexual partners and to their health caretakers. Ethics related to infectious diseases face problems induced by migration and the permeability of transnational borders to microorganisms unknown in host countries. The strong interdependence of poverty and susceptibility to infecting and transmitting agents needs to be taken into account in research and in eradication campaigns. Pharmaceutical industries' financial interest will often collide with the accessibility to medication and immunization in poor and distant regions. Biomedical research has systematically neglected the search for affordable vaccines against endemic diseases like malaria, and privately sponsored trials consistently support the 90:10 divide by preferably investing in marketable and profitable products. Not all infectious diseases are neglected. AIDS research has been lavishly funded and intensively pursued, no doubt because it is a very vivid threat to the well-being of the affluent.

More than other bioethics issues, infectious disease is intertwined with moral and religious considerations. Sexually transmitted diseases are related to promiscuity and unsafe sex; AIDS was initially believed to be a condition confined to homosexuals at a time when being gay was socially unacceptable and the Vatican made it publicly known that homosexual relations were sinful. Condoms were repeatedly rejected by the Catholic Church in Third World countries, under the predicament that they favoured casual sex, and public health was hampered in its efforts to control AIDS when the Church insisted that only abstinence is an adequate and morally acceptable protection.

5.2 Healthcare promotion

Health promotion is about convincing people to modify or adapt their habits and lifestyles in order to live healthy and disease free lives. Its basic tenet relies on stressing care and placing it at the same level of importance as cure. The explicit target of public health is to reduce population at risk, that is, the group or segment of the whole "which is making the greatest adverse contribution to the average" of a certain risk factor. The Canadian public approach has been to define a "Health Field Concept" that comprises four categories: human biology, environment, lifestyle, healthcare organization [Lalonde, 1981]. Such a very comprehensive public health strategy presents four *caveats*: First, sufficient resources should have secured adequate medical care services based on equal access; second, research ought to avoid excessive concentration on human biology –molecular epidemiology-, to the detriment of the other components of the health field concept; third, science has presented scanty and contradictory evidence concerning the causal impact of life-style factor, so that arguments intended to influence the public have not been convincing enough to significantly modify attitudes and habits; fourth, life-styles are negatively influenced by social determinants -urban stress, industrial pollution-, and by lavish and attractive campaigns to indulge in those habits that have been identified as health risks -alcohol consumption, fast cars, adventurous sports-. Health promotion faces complex situations that make observers wary whether resources are being judiciously and reasonably diverted from more pressing medical needs.

Public health will resort to promotional campaigns whenever it detects a health problem but sees no clear-cut way of solving it. Promoting healthcare has come to the forefront of medicine based on the prevalence of chronic, non-communicable diseases, the influence of risk factor epidemiology plagued by causal uncertainties, and the new public health's insistence on self-care. Disapproval ranges from behaviour patterns that people enjoy, to habits and practices they are unable to curtail, leading to disparate views on what well-being is about -exercise versus sedentary habits, diets versus gourmandising, abstinence versus indulging in recreational substances-. Especially in less affluent societies, health recommendations may be too onerous for the poor to follow.

Health promoting recommendations may reasonably revert to mandatory regulations when their effectiveness is proven beyond reasonable doubts, as in the mandatory use of seat-belts, alcohol-free driving, curtailment of passive smoking, vaccination as travel requirement. Unless it can be proven that certain practices are deleterious to others, or will adversely influence a public good, indications for healthy comportment remain bland and irregularly headed.

The effectiveness of promotional campaigns is anybody's guess. Social alcohol consumption may have harmful effects, but will hardly be influenced by deterrent campaigns. On the other hand, fads and fanaticism may be unleashed by persistent propaganda, and a state of protracted public panic may follow alarming official warnings or awesome media displays. Negative and uncertain consequences of promotional campaigns should be considered when planning allocation of scarce resources that will become unavailable for less spectacular but perhaps more basic healthcare needs.

5.3 Public health in war and bioterrorism

Armed conflicts have been an attractive intellectual turf for philosophy, especially in view of the 20th century's infamous record of two World Wars, ferocious regional conflicts, genocide, guerrilla warfare, and terrorism. Inevitably, bioethics has been involved in these matters, producing a considerable amount of literature where philosophical and ethical arguments are often polluted with military, political, doctrinal and other contingent considerations, thus stimulating harsh ideological discussions -"there is a rough symmetry between the underlying principles of contemporary just war and bioethics" [Gross, 2004]-, rather than deliberation and reasoned approaches.

The ethical reflection on armed conflicts revolves around the concepts of just war and the justification of acts of public violence. The doctrine of just war *-jus ad bellum-* accepts two circumstances as giving moral support to engage in armed hostilities in foreign territories: retaliation, and defending basic humanitarian principles that are being violated by rogue states. As for acceptable methods of warfare *-jus in bello-*, they explicitly disallow harming civilians and civilian targets, and engaging in exceptionally damaging aggressions such as biological and chemical arms. Torture has been condemned and prohibited, but unsettling allowances are made under the "ticking bomb" allegation, which purports the urgency of extracting information in order to avert major disasters [Lee, 2007].

The reason for bringing up these issues in a text on public health bioethics dates back to the 2002 terrorist attacks on New York. At that point, when terrorism threatened to be violating all restraints, fear of exacerbated bioterrorism was kindled by a few attempts at posting envelops with anthrax spores, leading officials and the media to engage public health in comprehensive programs including strategic preventive planning in the event of a terrorist induced epidemic, setting up emergency vaccination programs, as well as developing biological defensive and retaliatory weapons. The U.S. government responded with a huge allocation of resources to public health, alas 4/5th of which were earmarked for anti-bioterrorism research, the rest to support the precarious finances of routine public health programs.

Confident that public health had the expertise to deal with biological threats, the U.S. government called upon law scholars, officials and other experts to develop a Model State Emergency Health Power Act commissioned to design appropriate measures in case of catastrophic public health emergencies. Vaccination programs in strategic areas and for persons posing risks of massive contagion would be mandatory if needed; health officials would be empowered to regulate the distribution and pricing of scarce medical supplies, eventually compelling healthcare workers to remain on duty against their will [Hodge & Gostin, 2004]. Some scholars voiced their concern at the prospect of over-reactive precedents being set [Bayer & Colgrove, 2004], pointing out the perils of upsetting the delicate balance between individual rights and restrictive policies in order to secure protection of the public.

Many questions remained unanswered, anticipating havoc should bioterrorist emergencies occur in the future: ought chronically scarce public health resources to be used in research and policies concerned with biological terrorism? Who will set priorities in an emergency: military strategists or public health experts? How serious and imminent must a threat or an actual attack be to curtail rights and declare a state of emergency? Who will decide what commensurate and appropriate countermeasures to undertake?

In the final analysis, public health bioethics must feel unhappy when pragmatic and contingent arguments are employed to neglect and violate cherished moral standards and hard-won rights. Equally unsettling is the prospect that bioethics must be compelled to abide by the decisions of those in power when declaring a just war and allowing the arbitrary toleration of flagrantly abusive *jus in bello* practices - Guantánamo, Abu Ghraib-. Even though public health activities have historically been required to serve as the practical arm of political goals in form of medical police or biopolitics, current efforts at employing public health know-how for military purposes is a development that goes beyond what rational bioethics ought to justify.

6. Outlook

As for the future of public health, there is little information to allow educated guesses, and prognosis is mostly made from the vantage point of hopes and wishful thinking. Most people agree that health should be a right, to be universally claimed and honoured, which means including the marginalized, the poor, and the distant. But theory alone rarely transcends social realities, political vagaries, and economic pressures. Risk-factor epidemiology with its emphasis on the individual ought to be subordinated to population studies, focusing on socioeconomic and environmental conditions that need to be modified for the benefit of human health. The world is already enmeshed in deleterious influences on human populations´ health and survival conditions, requiring that present needs and interests be accounted for without neglecting the anticipated needs of future generations. Nevertheless, if resources are scarce, the future ought to be discounted in order to attend the pressing needs of the now living.

Propositions in ethics have a natural tendency to strongly collide with actual practices and trends. Risk factor epidemiology and the new public health are hostile to State protected human rights and deaf to healthcare as an obligation due to all and everyone. Market-oriented neoliberalism has little patience with strong, centrally planned and financed public health programs, and science prefers reductionist approaches and seductive technological developments, instead of searching for measures to solve grass-roots problems [Pearce, 1996]. These are widely differing and incompatible viewpoints, proving that bioethics in public health faces arduous work in deliberating these issues and enhancing a fundamental ethics protecting the common weal as widely and extensively as necessary. Public health is in permanent danger of becoming a puppet discipline of political forces and ideologies, unless it develops its own brand of applied bioethics engaged in exploring values and preferences that ought to inspire public health-related policies. This query will depend on fundamental political outlooks and reflection at the philosophical level, either understanding social factors as powerful forces capable of modelling and manipulating its citizens, or seeing human beings as individuals who freely structure their actions and their relations in a climate of secure social equity.

7. A wistful epilogue

History teaches that neither political power nor scientific discoveries triggering technical developments are the driving forces of public health. In fact, they seem to follow diverging pragmatic goals, often forgetting or unwilling to raise the question who the beneficiaries of these goals are or ought to be. Civilization and progress are no guarantees for a robust public health; quite to the contrary, material well-being leads neoliberal politics to neglect the public sphere and reduce the common weal to law and order. Much of public health's activities have been dictated by needs of the moment, above all catering to predominant vested interest. Reacting to emergencies or to pressing need is but one of public health's tasks, but a more fundamental question is its place in improving health standards and helping avoid diseases that can be eradicated, as well as mitigating such derangements as can be substantially reduced in their toll of suffering, poverty, disempowerment and premature death.

There are too many differing proposals to suggest that public health has found its way or is on the right path. There is little agreement about such basic concepts as health, disease, social commitment to primary prevention by central institutions, the need for publicly supported medical care, and the pursuance of relevant knowledge for meaningful and efficient health promotion. Should we understand health as well-being or as absence of disease? Shall disease be considered a predisposition, an overt derangement of the organism, a poor adaption to social and environmental conditions? Research in epidemiology wavers between molecular studies and analysis of social and economic contexts, because it remains an unsettled question whether health is better served by improving the world we live in, or seeking to increase individual defences and protection against external harshness that prevails beyond repair. These alternatives also trouble ecologists, illustrating how public health and the environment are intertwined in a common quest to better the human condition by making it less vulnerable and better adapted to thrive in the world it inhabits.

The obvious but self-defeating answer seems to be eclecticism served by interdisciplinary approaches, multicausal and multilevel explanations, and global proposals. Delaying pragmatic approaches while academia continues to delve in freely associative theorizing that eludes the knotty problems of reality, seems severely inadequate if we admit that by any standard or parameter, the human population is worse off than ever before: more poverty, hunger and endemic disease, increasing inequality in terms of material goods, and inequity in terms of justice. The environment is becoming unfriendly and future prospects are not promising.

Poverty and destitution affects billions of people. It has become standard procedure to introduce discussions on the woes of the world, by throwing in some impressive statistics about disease prevalence, hunger, poverty, and other dire deprivations. Such rhetoric should be employed sparingly, for it tends to anesthetize public opinion. The recognition of suffering is not a quantitative matter, it is more a question of emotional distress, moral uneasiness, and actual commitment. One might apply to statistics what S. Sontag wrote about the emotional dulling when permanently confronted with images of horror and suffering: "Shock can become familiar. As one can become habituated to horror in real life, one can become habituated to the horror of certain images." [Sontag, 2003]. If lively images can dull the senses, how much easier it is to become indifferent to sheer statistics that obscure the suffering of actual human beings.

Lamentations are usually followed by well-meant but unsubstantiated proposals that are too distant from *Realpolitik* -the realities of politics in a world dominated by economic reasoning-, to make any difference. Impotence fires the imagination, not always in a positive way: some voices consider that *status quo* conditions will lead to a Darwinian selection where the poor will not survive while the affluent make true their hopes of enhancement and post-human development. Dissent and concern must step down from the ivory tower and become involved in ample participative deliberation that emphasizes how moral legitimacy ought to precede legislation and political engagement.

There have been a few publications specifically addressing the "Philosophical basis for public health", that are exploring the field and coming up with some tentative suggestions to initiate a daunting task [Weed, 1999]. Bioethics in public health is called upon to deliberate in depth with the aim of emerging with reasonable proposals.

8. References

Almeida, C. (2002). Equidade e reforma sectorial na América Latina: um debate necessário. *Cadernos Saúde Pública* 18 (Supl), pp. (23-36)

Arouca, S. (2003). *O dilemma preventivista,* Editora UNESP-Editora FIOCRUZ, ISBN 85-72129-507-1, São Paulo – Rio de Janeiro.

Arras, J.D., Fenton E.M. (2009). Bioethics & human rights. *Hastings Center Report*, 39, pp. (17-38).

Battin, M. P, Smith, C.B., Francis, L.P., Jacobson, J.A. (2008). Towards control of infectious diseases: Ethical challenges for a global effort. In: *International public health policy and ethics*. Boylan, M. (ed.), pp. (191-214), Springer, ISBN 978-1-4020-8616-8, Dordrecht

Bayer, R., Colgrove J. (2004). Rights and dangers: bioterrorism and the ideologies of public health. In: *In the wake of terror*. Moreno, J.D. (ed.), pp. (51-74), The MIT Press, ISBN 0-262-63302-7, Cambridge London

Beauchamp, D.E., Steinbock, B. (1999). *New ethics for the public's health*, Oxford University Press, ISBN 0-19-512439-1, New York Oxford

Beauchamp, TL., Childress, JF. (2001). *Principles of biomedical ethics*. 5th ed. Oxford University Press, ISBN 0-19-514332-9, Oxford New York

Beaglehole, R. , Bonita, R. (1997). *Public health at the crossroads*, Cambridge University Press, ISBN 0 521 58665 8, Cambridge

Boylan, M. (2008). Introduction: international public health: morality, politics,poverty, war, disease. In: *International public health policy and ethics*, Boylan M. (ed.), pp. (1-12), Springer, ISBN 978-1-4020-8616-8, Dordrecht

Callon, M., Lascoumes, P., & Barthe, Y. (2001). *Agir dans un monde incertain*, Edition du Seuil, ISBN 978-2-02-040432-7, Paris

Caplan, A.L., Engelhardt Jr., H.T., & McCartney, J.J. (1981). *Concepts of health and disease*. Addison-Wesley Publishing Company, ISBN 0-201-00973-0-, Reading Mass.

Carrol, P.E. (2002). Medical police and the history of public health. *Medical History* 46, (461-494)

COMEST. (2005). *The precautionary principle*, UNESCO, Paris.

Cunnigham, A., Grell, O.P. (2000).*The four horsemen of the Apocalypse*, Cambridge University Press 2000. ISBN 0-521-46701-2, Cambridge UK

Daniels, N. (2006). Equity and population health: towards a broader bioethics agenda. *Hastings Center Report* 36, (22-35)

Daniels, N. (2008). International health inequalities and global justice. In: *International public health policy and ethics*, Boylan M. (ed.), pp. (109-129), Springer, ISBN 978-1-4020-8616-8, Dordrecht

Defoe, D. (1722) *A journal of the plague year*. Matsumoto T, Widger D. (Prod.) (2006). http://www.gutenberg.org Accessed Nov. 14, 2010

Dwyer, J. (2004). Illegal immigrants, healthcare, and social responsibility, *Hastings Center Report*, 34, pp. (34-41)

Dwyer, J. (2007). What's wrong with the global migration of healthcare professionals? Individual rights and international justice, *Hastings Center Report* 37 (36-43)

Fayerweather, W.E., Higginson, J., Beauchamp, T.L. (eds.) (1991). Ethics in epidemiology. *Journal of Clinical Epidemiology* 44, Supp. I, (1S-170S)

Fraser N. *Scales of justice*. (2009). Columbia University Press, ISBN 978-0-231-14680-7, New York

Goddard O. (2001). Principe de Précaution. In: *Nouvelle encyclopédie de bioéthique*, Hottois G, Missa J-N. (eds.), pp. (650-658), De Boeck Université, ISBN 2-8041-3712-0, Bruxelles

Goldstein, B.D. (2001). The precautionary principle also applied to public health actions. *American Journal of Public Health*, 91, 9, pp. (1358-1361)

Gordon, J.S. (2008). Poverty, human rights, and just distribution. In: *International public health policy and ethics*, Boylan, M. (ed.), , pp. (131-141), Springer, ISBN 978-1-4020-8616-8, Dordrecht

Gostin, L. (2002). Public health law, ethics, and human rights: mapping the issues. In: *Public Health law and ethics: a reader,* Gostin L (ed.), University of California Press: 1-19. ISBN 0-520-23174-9, Berkeley Los Angeles*The Milbank Quarterly*, 88, pp. (149-168)

Gross, M. (2004). *Bioethics and armed conflict*, The MIT Press, ISBN 0-262-57226-5-, Cambridge London

Hedgecoe, A.M. (2004). Critical bioethics: science critique of applied ethics. *Bioethics,* 18, pp. (102-143)

Harris, J. (2007). *Enhancing evolution*, Princeton University Press, ISBN 978-0-691-12844, Princeton Oxford

Hessler, K. (2008). Exploring the philosophical foundations of the human rights approach to international public health ethics. In: *International public health policy and ethics,* Boylan M. (ed.), pp. (31-43), Springer, ISBN 978-1-4020-8616-8, Dordrecht

Hobbes, T. (1978). Leviathan (1651), Collins/Fontana, ISBN 0 00 633066 5, Glasgow

Hodge Jr., J.G., Gostin, L.O. (2004). Protecting the public's health in an era of bioterrorism: the Model State Emergency Health Power Act. In: *In the wake of terror*, Moreno JD. (ed.), pp. (17-32) The MIT Press, ISBN 0-262-63302-7, Cambridge London

Illies, C. (2008) Why should we help the poor? Philosophy and poverty. In: *International public health policy and ethics,* Boylan M. (ed.), pp. (143-156), Springer, ISBN 978-1-4020-8616-8, Dordrecht

Kass, N.E. (2001). An ethics framework for public health. *American Journal of Public Health* 91, pp. (1776-1782)

Kriebel, D. & Tickner, J. (2001). Reenergizing public health through precaution. *American Journal of Public Health,* 91, 9, pp. (1351-1355)

Krieger, N. (1999). Questioning epidemiology: objectivity, advocacy, and socially responsible science. *American Journal of Public Health,* 89, 8, pp. (1151-1153)

Lalonde M. (1981). *A new perspective on the health of Canadians*. Minister of Supply and Services Canada. ISBN 0-661-50019-9, Ottawa

Lee SP. (2007). *Intervention, terrorism, and torture,* Springer, ISBN 2-4020-4677-4, Dordrecht

Lloyd GER. (1978). *Hippocratic writings*. Harmondsworth, Penguin Books Ltd. ISBN 0 14 040.031 1.

Macey D. (2009).Rethinking biopolitics, race and power in the wake of Foucault. *Theory, Culture & Society* 6:186-205.

Mann JM. (1997). Medicine and Public Health. Ethics and Human Rights. *Hastings Center Report* 27, pp. (6-13)

Marchant GE. (2003). From general policy to legal rule: aspirations and limitations of the precautionary principle. *Environmental Health Perspectives* 14, pp. (1799-1803)

Mechanic D. (1978). Medical sociology, The Free Press, ISBN 0-02-920720-7, New York
Nozick R. (1974). Anarchy, state and utopia, Basic books ISBN 0 631 19780 X, New York
Nussbaum, M. (2006). *Frontiers of justice.* Cambridge, The Belknap Press, ISBN 0-674-01917-2, London
O'Neill, O. (1998).*Towards justice and virtue*, Cambridge University Press. ISBN 0 521 48099 2, Cambridge
Pearce, N. (1996). Traditional epidemiology, modern epidemiology, and public health, *Amercian Journal Public Health* 86, pp. (678-683)
Petersen, A., Lupton, D. (2000). *The new public health.* Sage Publications, ISBN 0 7619 5404, London
Petryna, A. (2007). Clinical trials offshored: on private sector science and public health. *BioSocieties* 2, pp. (21-40),London
Pogge, T.W. (2005). *World poverty and human rights.* Cambridge UK, Polity Press, ISBN 0-7456-2995-4-
Purdy, L. (2004). The politics of preventing premature death. In: *Public health policy and ethics*, Boylan M. (ed.), pp. (167-185), Kluwer Academic Publisher. ISBN 1-4020-1763-4, Dordrecht.
Purdy L. (2008). Exporting the "Culture of Life". In *International public health policy and ethics*, Boylan, M. (ed.), pp. (91-106), Springer: ISBN 978-1-4020-8616-8, Dordrecht
Quigley, M., Harris, J. (2008). Personal or public health? In: *International public health policy and ethics,* Boylan M. (ed.), pp. (15-29), Springer, ISBN 978-1-4020-8616-8, Dordrecht
Rothman D. (1991). *Strangers at the bedside.* Basic Books. ISBN 0-465-08210-6.
Rose, G. (1985). Sick individuals and sick population. *International Journal of Epidemiology* 14, pp. 32- 38.
Rosen, G. (1993). *A history of public health.* The Johns Hopkins University Press. ISBN 0-8018-4645-5, Baltimore
Selgelid, M.J. (2005). Ethics and infectious disease. *Bioethics* 2005;19:272-289.
Sen, A. (1995). *Inequality reexamined.* Harvard University Press. ISBN 0-674-45256-9, Cambridge Mass.
Sen, A. (2000). *Development as freedom*. New YoeK; Alfred A. Knopf. ISBN 0-375-40619-0.
Singer, P. (2004). Outsiders: our obligation to those beyond our borders. In: *The ethics of assistance,* Chatterjee D. (ed.), pp. (11-32), Cambridge University Press, ISBN 0 521 52742 2, Cambridge UK
Sontag S. (2003). *Regarding the pain of others.* Picador, ISBN 0-312-42219-9, New York
Susser, M. (1998). Does risk factor epidemiology put epidemiology at risk? Peering into the future. *Journal of Epidemiology & Community Health* 52, pp. (608-611)
Susser, M., Susser, E. (1996). Choosing a future for epidemiology: from black box to Chinese boxes and eco-epidemiology. *American Journal Public Health* 86, pp. (825-829)
Starfield, B., Hyde, Jj, & Gervas, J., Heath I. (2008). The concept of prevention: a good idea gone astray. *Journal of Epidemiology & Community Health* 62, pp. (580-583)
Touraine, A. (1985). An introduction to the study of social movements. *Social Research* 52, pp. (749-787)

Van der Maesen, L.J.G., Nijhuis H.G.J. (2000). Continuing the debate on the philosophy of modern public health: social quality as a point of reference. *Journal of Epidemiology & Community Health* 54, (134-142)

Verweij, M., Dawson, A. (2007).The meaning of 'public' in 'public health'. In: *Ethics, prevention and public health,* Dawson, A., Verweij, M. (eds.). (2007). Oxford University Press, ISBN 978-0-19-929069-7, Oxford.

Victora, C.G., Habicht, J-P., & Bryce, J. (2004). Evidence-based public health: Moving beyond randomized trials. *American Journal of Public Health* 94, pp. (400-405)

Weed, D.L. (1999). Towards a philosophy of public health. *Journal of Epidemiology & Community Health* 53, pp. (99-104)

Weed D.L. &, McKeown,R.E. (2003). Science and social responsibility in public health. *Environmental Health Perspectives,* 111, 14, pp. (1804-1818)

6

Adolescence - A New Multilevel Approach on the HIV/AIDS Patient

Largu Maria Alexandra, Manciuc Doina Carmen and Dorobăţ Carmen
The Infectious Diseases Hospital Iaşi, Romania

1. Introduction

This paper derives from a series of attempts to study not only the medical characteristics of the HIV infected population in the Moldova area of Romania, but also the psychological aspects that are undeniably linked to them. For the past 22 years (since the fall of the communist regime) the Romanian population has been made aware of the existence of HIV in our country, has been educated in terms of the specific aspects of this infection, and has recently been a target for strong campaigns against discrimination and stigma. All these aspects make up the social background in which HIV infected children, adolescents and adults evolve.

The main population of HIV positives in our country is made op of a specific age group, due to a mass infection in the early 1990's, in children's hospitals. So now we address mostly adolescents and young people who are known to be infected for 20 or more years.

The authors' aim in this paper is to describe the unique characteristics that adolescence imposes, as an important age group, in terms of the specific features reflected on the HIV/AIDS patient. This is important because adolescence is defined by a series of processes that finalize in contouring the human mind and defining the personality. Although nothing is fully stable and permanent, and personality can suffer changes in time, adolescence leaves a decisive mark on the way different personality traits and psychological processes manifest themselves.

Also, the specific elements that define the mental and emotional development of the HIV patient determine a certain direction in contouring the adolescent's personality.

That is why we consider that there is need for a certain medical, social and psychological approach to this age group, regarding infected patients. The importance of studying the interaction of these variables is strongly reflected in the improvement of everyday practices in medical and care institutions, as well as in the social perception of HIV infected people (although this is a field in which education is continuous). Informing people about certain issues that have been, until recently, considered "taboo", can be a step in combating discrimination, which would enable the young people in the category we address to effectively insert themselves in society and to have a smooth and complete social, professional, and emotional development.

2. The HIV positive adolescent

In this chapter we will attempt to describe the main characteristics of the HIV/AIDS infection from a medical and social point of view. We will also detail the most important features of the HIV/AIDS infected person aged 16 to 22.

2.1 The HIV infection

The infection with the human immunodeficiency virus (HIV) in its most advanced stage, also known as the acquired immunodeficiency syndrome (AIDS) is characterized clinically by a complex and predominantly cellular immune deficiency, which predisposes to various other infections: bacterial, viral, fungal, protozoal, with invariably fatal developments in months or years. The HIV infection causes a collapse in the CD4 immune defense system, central nervous system infections, opportunistic infections and the emergence of tumors.
The causal agent is the HIV retrovirus, which only affects the CD4 receptor-LT4 cells, tissue and neurons, and multiply in the presence of antibodies.

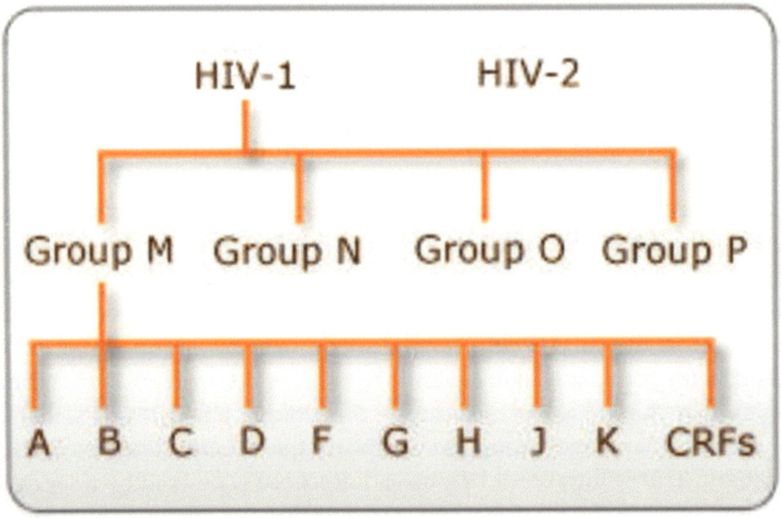

Fig. 1. The different types of HIV

There are two known strand of HIV. HIV-1 was first described in 1983 by Luc Montagnier, followed in 1984 by Le Gallo. In 1986 HIV-2 was also identified.
The transmission of this retrovirus is done directly - sexually, through blood, intrauterine - or indirectly - through the use of infected syringes by drug abusers, from mother to child during birth, or unsterilized medical instruments. Risk groups most affected are male homo / heterosexuals, hemophiliacs, people who have heterosexual relations with multiple partners, blood transfusion recipients, newborns whose mothers are HIV positive.
There are six developmental stages of the virus: incubation, infection, symptomatic infection, generalized lymphadenopathy, ARC (AIDS Related Complex), AIDS.
Incubation (1) extends over a period of 1-3 months, and the asymptomatic or sexual infection (2) 10 to 14 months. Antibodies appear 6-12 weeks after infection. In stage 3 – the symptomatic infection – neurological, liver and skin symptoms are present. Stage 4, the generalized limphadenopathy is the stage where at least three ganglion groups are

identified, during a period of over three months. They are evidence of the efforts the immune system makes to fight the pathogen that entered the body. Stage 5 - ARC (AIDS Related Complex) is characterized by a remarkable weight loss and the presence of fever for more than a month. In the last stage - AIDS - opportunistic infections and tumors are already present.

According to the AVERT up to date information, there are four known strains o HIV-1. They can be classified into four groups: the "major" group M, the "outlier" group O and two new groups, N and P. These four groups may represent four separate introductions of simian immunodeficiency virus into humans.

Group O appears to be restricted to west-central Africa and group N - a strain discovered in 1998 in Cameroon - is extremely rare. In 2009 a new strain closely relating to gorilla simian immunodeficiency virus was discovered in a Cameroonian woman. It was designated HIV-1 group P. More than 90% of HIV-1 infections belong to HIV-1 group M and, unless specified, the rest of this page will relate to HIV-1 group M only.

Within group M there are known to be at least nine genetically distinct subtypes (or clades) of HIV-1. These are subtypes A, B, C, D, F, G, H, J and K.

Occasionally, two viruses of different subtypes can meet in the cell of an infected person and mix together their genetic material to create a new hybrid virus (a process similar to sexual reproduction, and sometimes called "viral sex"). Many of these new strains do not survive for long, but those that infect more than one person are known as "circulating recombinant forms" or CRFs. For example, the CRF A/B is a mixture of subtypes A and B.

One of the CRFs is called A/E because it is thought to have resulted from hybridization between subtype A and some other "parent" subtype E. However, no one has ever found a pure form of subtype E. Confusingly, many people still refer to the CRF A/E as "subtype E" (in fact it is most correctly called CRF01_AE).

A virus isolated in Cyprus was originally placed in a new subtype I, before being reclassified as a recombinant form A/G/I. It is now thought that this virus represents an even more complex CRF comprised of subtypes A, G, H, K and unclassified regions. The designation "I" is no longer used.

The HIV-1 subtypes and CRFs are typically associated with certain geographical regions, with the most widespread being subtypes A and C. As studies have shown, individuals are increasingly presenting with sub-types not native to the country of diagnosis. For example, a rise of non-B sub-types among men who have sex with men (MSM) in the UK has been identified.

Subtype A and CRF A/G predominate in West and Central Africa, with subtype A possibly also causing much of the Russian epidemic.

Historically, subtype B has been the most common subtype/CRF in Europe, the Americas, Japan and Australia and is the predominant sub-type found among MSM infected in Europe. Although this remains the case, other subtypes are becoming more frequent and now account for at least 25% of new HIV infections in Europe.

Subtype C is predominant in Southern and East Africa, India and Nepal. It has caused the world's worst HIV epidemics and is responsible for around half of all infections.

Subtype D is generally limited to East and Central Africa.

A subtype E has not been isolated. However, CRF A/E is prevalent in South-East Asia, but originated in Central Africa.

Subtype F has been found in Central Africa, South America and Eastern Europe.

Subtype G and CRF A/G have been observed in West and East Africa and Central Europe. Subtype H has only been found in Central Africa; J only in Central America; and K only in the Democratic Republic of Congo and Cameroon.

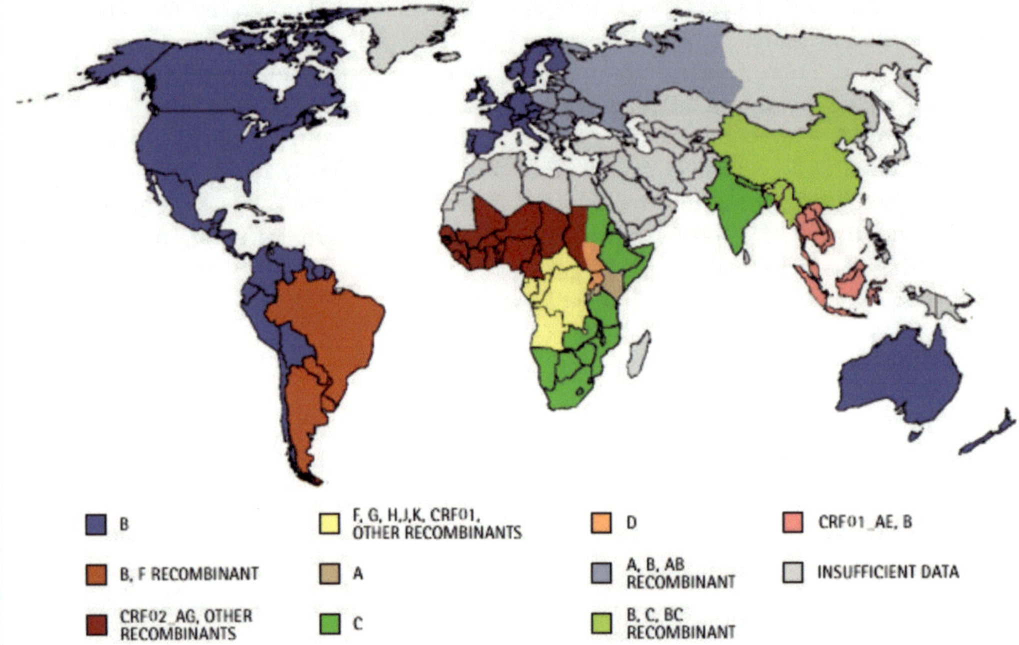

Fig. 2. HIV Subtypes around the world

A study presented in 2006 found that Ugandans infected with subtype D or recombinant strains incorporating subtype D developed AIDS sooner than those infected with subtype A, and also died sooner, if they did not receive antiretroviral treatment. The study's authors suggested that subtype D is more virulent because it is more effective at binding to immune cells. This result was supported by another study presented in 2007, which found that Kenyan women infected with subtype D had more than twice the risk of death over six years compared with those infected with subtype A. An earlier study of sex workers in Senegal, published in 1999, found that women infected with subtype C, D or G were more likely to develop AIDS within five years of infection than those infected with subtype A. Several studies conducted in Thailand suggest that people infected with CRF A/E progress faster to AIDS and death than those infected with subtype B, if they do not receive antiretroviral treatment.

The main subtype found in Romania is F, whit a very long life span, of over 20 years with proper antiretroviral treatment.

Detection of specific anti-HIV antibodies is done by two methods: ELISA and Western Blott test. Negative results from these tests indicate the absence of infection, while positive results mark the presence of HIV in the blood. These tests can sometimes be negative in infected people, due to the presence of an immunological window of 6-12 weeks (corresponding to the incubation period).

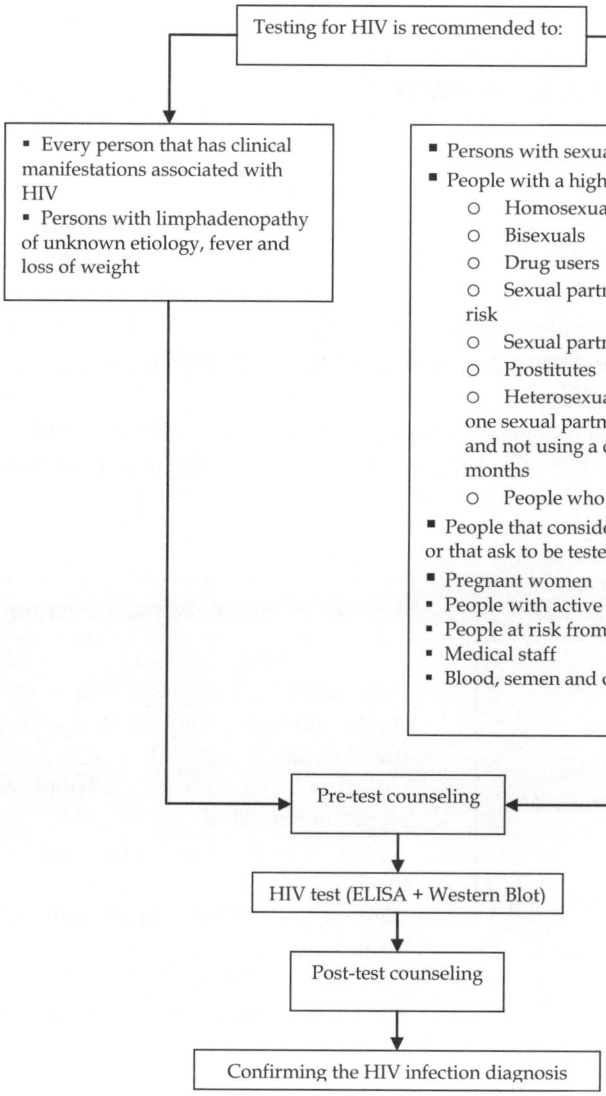

Fig. 3. The algorithm for HIV testing

Pre- and post-test counseling is first of all based on the principle of confidentiality, which establishes a trusting connection between the counselor and the patient. There are two main goals in counseling, and these are: 1. preventing the transmission of the HIV infection; 2. socially and psychologically supporting people who have been infected. The most important aspects covered by counseling in the case of HIV/AIDS are:

- supplying information about the HIV infection:
  - what the HIV infection is and how it evolves
  - ways of transmission and ways of prevention
  - diagnosis: the meaning of a negative, undetermined or positive test
- determining the risk factor of a person's behavior
- helping the person understand and admit the risks certain behaviors pose

- defining the degree of specificity that a certain behavior has for the person's life style
- helping the person find resources to eliminate a risky behavior
- supporting the person in any positive change

Once the infection detected, the patient is advised and informed about the importance of adherence to therapy. Medication prevents the spread of HIV in the blood, helps support the immune system, and thus prolongs the patient's life considerably.

There are currently more than 20 approved antiretroviral drugs in the US and Europe (including combined formulations) and many more in the expanded access programs and trials. Like most medicines, antiretroviral drugs can cause side effects. These unwanted effects are often mild, but sometimes they are more serious and can have a major impact on health or quality of life. On rare occasions, side effects can be life threatening.

Once started, antiretroviral treatment must be taken every day for life. Every missed dose increases the risk that the drugs will stop working. It is therefore vital that people receiving antiretroviral treatment get all the help they need to minimize the impact of side effects. Often there are several ways to lessen the harm, either by treating the side effects or by switching to alternative antiretroviral drugs.

Symptom	Drug used	Advice on how to reduce the symptom
Diarrhea	Especially protease inhibitors	- Eat less insoluble fiber (raw vegetables, fruit skins, wholegrain bread or cereal, seeds and nuts) and replace with soluble fiber (white rice, pasta) - Cut down on caffeine, alcohol and the sweetener sorbitol - Avoid greasy, fatty, spicy and sugary foods - Reduce dairy products in case of lactose intolerance - Consult a dietician
Nausea and vomiting	Almost all antiretroviral drugs	- Eat several small meals instead of a few large meals - Avoid spicy, greasy and rich foods; choose bland foods - Eat cold rather than hot meals - Don't drink with a meal or soon after - Avoid alcohol, aspirin and smoking - Avoid cooking smells
Rash	Nevirapine, abacavir	- Avoiding hot showers or baths - Using milder toiletries and laundry detergents - Wearing cool fibers such as cotton, and avoiding wool - Humidifying the air - Trying moisturizers/emollients or calamine lotion

Lipodystrophy	Combinations of drugs from the NRTI and protease inhibitor classes	Switching antiretroviral treatment should stop the symptoms getting worse, but is unlikely to lead to much improvement once the condition has advanced.
Lipid abnormalities that cause heart conditions	Combinations of drugs from the NRTI and protease inhibitor classes	- Give up smoking - Take more exercise - Cut calories and eat less fat - Consume more fibers and omega-3 fatty acids

Table 1. Main types of side effects

Side effects vary from person to person and it is impossible to predict exactly how each individual will be affected. Some people take antiretroviral treatment for years with few problems, while others find the same drugs intolerable. Nevertheless some characteristics and pre-existing conditions (such as high blood pressure or hepatitis infection) are known to increase the risk from certain side effects. Doctors should assess these factors before advising patients on which drugs to choose.

Some side effects appear shortly after starting an antiretroviral drug and disappear within a few weeks as the body gets used to the new chemicals. This is often the case with nausea, diarrhea and headache, for example.

Unfortunately other side effects - such as peripheral neuropathy (nerve damage) and lipodystrophy (fat redistribution) - tend to worsen over time and may never go away. Also some problems may not emerge until months or even years after treatment is started.

The main feature of patients living with HIV in Romania is that they are part of a large cohort representing almost 90% of children born during 1988-1989. These patients were diagnosed with HIV infection at the age of 3-6 years and have lived with HIV entire period of childhood and adolescence, being supervised and monitored by both families and medical staff of the infectious diseases clinics. Therefore they have grown along side the development of therapeutic lines, while passing from mono- and bi-therapy to HAART therapy. Many of them have over 10 experimental regimens, including the use of the latest generation of protease inhibitors and coformulations of nucleoside inhibitors. Another specific feature for these patients is the coinfection with hepatitis B and C in over 12% of all cases. The delta strand of the hepatitis virus is also present, 1% of all HIV/AIDS adolescents suffering from a hepatitis B + D + C coinfection.

2.2 Social aspects of HIV/AIDS

Jonathan Mann, former Director of the Global HIV/AIDS of World Health Organization, made reference, in 1987, to three major HIV-related global epidemics.

The first concerns the epidemic of the HIV infection, which enters silently and unnoticed in the community as the infected person may not be aware of it throughout the incubation period and even in the asymptomatic infection.

The second is the AIDS epidemic, which occurs when the HIV infection causes serious disease - when a pathogen enters the body and the immune system can not cope, resulting in severe immunological collapse and all the symptoms previously described.

The third component is the social, cultural, economic and political, response given to the first two types of epidemics. "The sociological and epidemiological research on the AIDS phenomenon focuses on the dimensions and implications of socio-cultural, demographic, economic and political aspects of this complex phenomenon, which began as a medical problem, and became in time a real and disturbing social problem." (Buzducea, 1997) It is linked to discrimination, stigma, blaming, collective rejecting, which prevents an effective fight against the first two types of epidemics.

In her paper published in 2003, Doina Usaci made a survey of public attitudes towards the threat of AIDS. She stresses out that behavioral and attitude responses reflect a gap between the four plans addressing the phenomenon: cognitive, affective, behavioral and attitudinal. Each of these plans is marked, in turn, by the internal contradictions and ambivalent tendencies, which confirm an inadequacy of psychological responses in relation to the magnitude of the epidemic.

The cognitive plan is ahead of the other plans in terms of its development, as proven by a good level of knowledge regarding ways of transmission of the virus and ways of protection. But it is burdened by conflicting issues and ambivalent trends, rendering it inoperable in terms of the person's inner state.

The affective plan prevails over the cognitive in terms of maintaining inner balance. Fear is the dominant emotion, distorting perception and risk assessment, in the sense of over-evaluating it – up to reactions of phobic avoidance of sexual relations - or undermining its importance, as a result of the maladaptive action of defense mechanisms such as denial or rationalization, designed to reduce anxiety.

From a behavioral point of view, the author identifies ambivalent trends regarding the option for certain protective strategies, and an obvious gap between intention and act in terms of their implementation.

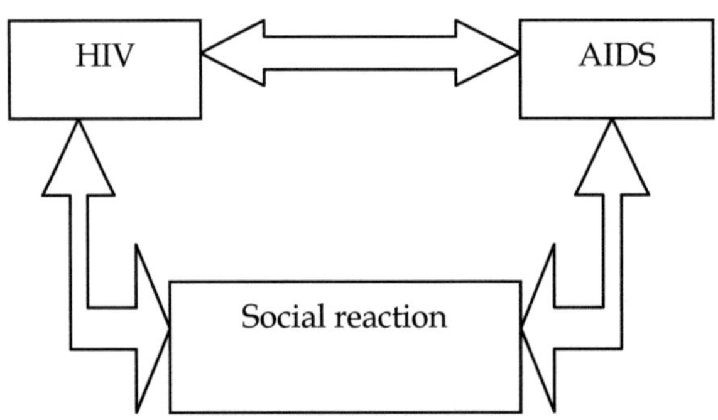

Fig. 4. The interaction between the three types of epidemics

The attitude plan is itself encumbered by striking internal contradictions, with mostly social effects. Attitudes towards infected people are ambivalent, oscillating between solidarity and distance, even rejection and guilt.

The author concludes that HIV/AIDS infection-related issues define an "irrational" conduct in relation to the magnitude of the epidemic and the dangers of social division which it hides.
"Stigma, silence, discrimination and rejection, as well as breaches in confidentiality, damage all efforts of prevention, care, treatment, and increase the impact of the AIDS epidemic on individuals, families, communities and nations." United Nations Declaration of Commitment on HIV/AIDS

2.3 Growing up with HIV/AIDS – the main characteristics of the Infected child and adolescent

Kristin Close (2007) presented data that highlighted the prevalence of HIV in the population under 15 years. Thus, in 2007, approximately 2.1 million children under 15 were living with HIV, and the same year 290 000 children died due to infection.
In Romania, more than two thirds of HIV the infected population consists of adolescents. Most were infected in the first years of life through unscreened blood transfusions. They are innocent victims of the pandemic. An impressive number of them have been abandoned in orphanages because of parental ignorance, poor living conditions or other disabilities associated with the disease. The rest remained in the family, where they had essentially two distinct types of attitudes: acceptance and support, or blame and stigma - according to their parents' education level and understanding of the disease (Buzducea, 1997).
In her paper Kristin Close (2007) describes the three main stages from childhood to adult stage. Pre-adolescence is described as a period of change in preferences, in terms of re-orientating attachment from parents and care-givers to fellow peers. Adolescence itself is predominantly marked by building self-image and abstract thinking. Late adolescence is the period of equilibrium, in which young people begin to feel comfortable with that identity and develop a social framework.
HIV infected people face a number of obstacles in addition to completing these steps.
One major consequence of ineffective treatment or late identification of the disease is poor physical development, along with impaired neurological and psychological development. Even if the proper treatment is established, taking it may have serious end often visible side effects, as listed above
Dislipidemy, for example, is a metabolic anomaly of plasmatic lipids and lipoproteins with a high risk of coronary disease, and it is very important in the development of HIV patients. Affecting the distribution of fat throughout the person's body is one of the most obvious and easily noticeable symptoms of this condition. In the case of a child or a teenager, this may affect their body image, as well as the way they are perceived by others.
Any physical condition is sure to mark the adolescence period and may cause difficulty in identifying with persons of the same age. This in turn affects the person's chances to interact with peers and get close to someone, thus forming meaningful relationships. Since personal identity emerges by comparing with others, young people aware of their HIV positive status may have a more negative self-image, may feel inferior, especially in the presence of social stigma.
Adolescence is also a period of exploration of oneself and the social environment. The stress of living with a chronic illness, such as AIDS, can prevent young people in taking any exploratory steps, or any initiatives that they should normally have. Living with AIDS

implies facing a number of challenges that shape identity, leading to a particular perspective on the world.

3. Realities faced by HIV-positives

In this third part of our paper we will present two relevant studies that underline the feelings HIV/AIDS patients have towards discrimination and the attitudes they come across every day. We will also describe a particular group of HIV infected adolescents, the residents of the "Gulliver" Hospice Placement Center.

3.1 Discrimination

A very important problem in the complex area of social interactions derives from every individual's unique way of being. Each person is different from every one else of its kind, even though we are all similar in a fundamental manner. It is this uniqueness that makes interactions dynamic and challenging, but it is also the basis of a rejection process, that targets everything that is too uncommon. Two words come to mind when dealing with this phenomenon - discrimination and stigmatization.

According to the Romanian Dictionary, "discrimination" is defined as a politic in which a certain country or group of citizens are deprived of certain rights, on an unfounded basis, and "stigmatization" is the casting on someone of public disgust, the feverishly condemnation of someone to dishonor.

Seen as a problem of interest for society as a whole, psychologists have tried to find the roots of the discrimination phenomena. The most pertinent conclusion is that discrimination comes from childhood, from our education, and it is founded on many generations of prejudice. It is hard for us to think flexibly because we are educated in a manner that encourages classifications. Everything has to be "put into boxes" and "stored on shelves", which makes us have a good perspective on things, but not on people. One tends to judge appearances more than essence, and so each individual is depersonalized, classified according to one feature or aspect that is relevant to the classifier. So one often ignores what people really are, overseeing real value. In order to rid ourselves of this highly indoctrinating way of thinking, we are in desperate need to open ourselves to the new.

The Romanian law system forbids discrimination in terms of race, nationality, ethnic or social background, sex or sexual orientation, or any other criteria that may restrain or stop the use of equality, human rights, or fundamental freedoms, politically, economically, socially, culturally or in any other public area. But discrimination exists! A survey made by Metro Media Transylvania - Barometrul de opinie privind discriminarea în România - 2004 shows that our country has high levels of discrimination against women, elderly people, poor people, national minorities, sexual minorities and HIV/AIDS infected people.

National minorities, sexual minorities, people with a low social status, have all been discriminated against for a long time, and the discrimination has been fought rigorously. As for HIV/AIDS patients, the disease and all the phenomena it causes are relatively new.

An online survey by the „Deschideți inima" ("Open Your Heart") organization posed this question: "How frequent do you think discrimination against HIV/AIDS infected people in Romania is?" The results were that the majority of people who answered believe that discrimination is "Very Frequent" (53.55%) or "Frequent" (34.04%). This proves that people are well aware of discriminating attitudes towards themselves or other people.

For the HIV infected person, discrimination manifests itself every day, through the interactions with different people - a neighbor, a friend, or former friend, even a relative. Coming across phrases like: "I can't shake hands with you."; "You're not my son anymore.", "Leave my street!" becomes a daily routine. Finding rejection where there was once trust and understanding is one of the main aspects people fear when they find that their HIV result came out positive. All the attitudes of people around a patient have a huge impact on his mental state, affecting self-esteem, as well as compliance to therapy, performances in life, and the ability to interact with others.

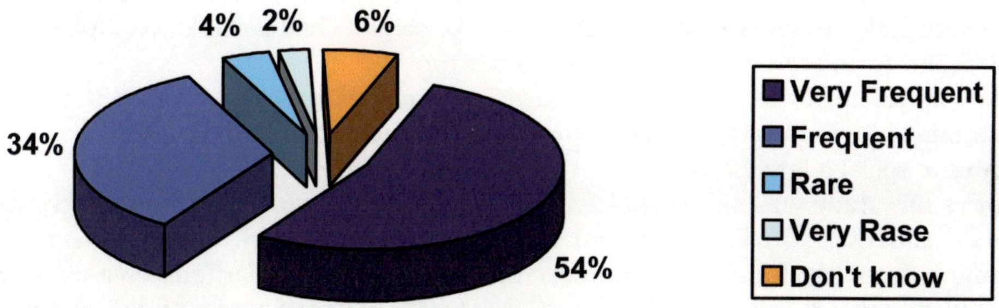

Fig. 5. The distribution of answers to the online survey made by „Deschideţi inima" ("Open Your Heart")

In 2008 the Regional Center for HIV/AIDS Iaşi conducted a study aimed to evaluate the degree of discrimination felt by the HIV infected patient in every-day social interactions.
100 patients assisted by the regional HIV/AIDS centre were tested using the clinical interview. Of these, 58 were male and 42 female, 32% from the rural area and 68% form the urban area. The average age was 20.9 years. The subjects had an average of 6 grades, with extremes from 4 grades to upper education. While 70% came from normal families, 20% had dysfunctional families and 10 % came from foster care. Of these, only 12% had a stabile job, 88% being unemployed.
Patients were encouraged to speak freely about the way in which informing others about their HIV status caused a change in attitude. Psychologists used a series of questions meant to pinpoint discrimination at the work place, in families, in groups of friends, as well as in other social contexts. One particular question - "Do you believe that the people around you who don't know you are infected would see you differently if they found out?" - was meant to reveal the patients expectations on other people's reactions, based on their experience.
The clinical interview revealed that 75% of all patients felt discriminated against, due to being infected with HIV.

3.2 An adolescent's view on social stigma

As stated earlier, growing up with a life long chronic condition such as AIDS has a strong impact in the physical, mental, emotional, as well as social development of an adolescent. The specific features of the post-communist society in Romania gives this struggle a whole new dimension, due to people's fear, lack of information and

A similar study was conducted in 2009, also in the HIV/AIDS Regional Center in Iaşi. It targeted the particular way in which HIV infected adolescents assisted by the Center perceived discrimination and/or the support of their social environment.

The study included 200 HIV/AIDS infected patients, who were asked to answer a series of questions devised by the team of psychologist from the Iaşi Regional Center. They also took part in a clinical interview and focus groups.

The majority of patients were male (59%), with an average age of 21.1 years. 66% came from an urban environment. As for schooling, the average level was 6 grades, with extremes between 2 classes and higher education. 14% of patients had a stable work place at that time. 38% came form broken up families or foster care.

The clinical interview, as well as the questionnaires, revealed that 83% of patients feel marginalized in society, due to being infected, and most of them (92%) try to hide their status in social interactions.

For us this study was important because it made clear the fact that the altered perception of HIV-positives in social relations and work, the low school level, as well as their background, coming from dysfunctional families, makes these particular adolescents a vulnerable population that requires an ethical approach from a series of angles and disciplines.

3.3 Orphans living with HIV/AIDS – case study on the young people in the "Gulliver" hospice placement center

The "Gulliver" placement center is a hospice-type care institution. It provides shelter for approximately 40 HIV positive young people, which have been abandoned at birth. The institution was established in the early 1990s, a time when Romania faced an outbreak of HIV. Fear and lack of knowledge led families

D. Bowlby called the personality type of a baby abandoned at birth "character without emotion." The most important traits of this specific type are: intellectual retardation, failure to establish deep relationships with others, low emotional reactions, aggression, low self-confidence, heightened by antisocial trends that are closely linked to emotional problems - even smiling and crying are affected and less representative for genuine emotions. Records also report tantrums, hyperactivity, and passiveness, extreme levels of apathy and in some cases going as far as autism. Even the relatively well-integrated and apparently balanced children encounter difficulties in developing authentic feelings and in establishing social contacts. Family abandonment is the main act that marks the abandoned personality. The effects of early psycho-trauma are undeniable and they mark the whole socio-psycho-emotional development of children.

Institutionalization is considered by the state to be a temporary solution, especially for what experts call either family failure or its vulnerability or inability to provide care and education. However, the social and economic situation in Romania determines a large number of families to consider placing their children in an orphanage.

Care institutions accommodate children to continuous exposure, excessive control, and poor relationships with significant adults, away from natural backgrounds such as family and

wider social community. Constant exposure limits the child and future adolescent's possibility to relax and engage in activities to release tension.
A recent study conducted in November 2002 showed that 50% of Romanian people believe that young people leaving placement centers do not have a real chance of integration into society when they come of age.
Young people, in their desire to integrate into the system, must cope and deal with a number of instances of socialization and control. Marginalization of youth stems from a limitation of their orientation to social work. Their situation is thus characterized by the absence of mechanisms that allow them to govern their own existence. Most often, marginalization leads to antisocial behavior, accompanied by school neglect, indifference to social norms, alcohol and drugs, physical and verbal aggression.
To all the psychological and social difficulties that young people growing up in orphanages face, the HIV / AIDS status adds an even greater burden, that of being labeled and rejected. Adolescents deal with their peers' fear of the disease, which translates into a fear of the person carrying the disease.
Marginalization of the HIV-positive young people, more so those coming from placement centers, feeds their the inability to achieve long term objectives, like adherence to the ARV treatment, finding a job, supporting themselves, developing meaningful relationships with the opposite sex.

4. The management of the HIV-infected adolescent

The HIV/AIDS patient has a number of features that need to be addressed in a specific manner. It is important to focus on three major targets - biological, social and psychological - when dealing with this particular type of patient. The biological target is usually set by the infectious diseases doctor and it involves mainly the personal effort of the patient. The social and psychological targets, however, are set by the patient and the psychologist and social worker who assist him in finding his balance and evolving in society. These two targets are destined not only for the patient, but also for the community in which he lives, that needs to undergo changes in order to accommodate him.

4.1 The biological target in addressing the HIV/AIDS adolescent

The first target is the biological aspect of a patient's treatment. The objectives in this case can be discussed from a clinical, virusological and immunological point of view.
The main clinical objective is to prologue the patient's life span and to improve his quality of life.
The virusological objective is to reduce the viral load as much as possible, preferably under 20 copies/ml and for a long period of time. This is a key factor in stopping or slowing down the progression of the disease, and also in preventing or delaying the appearance of resistant strands.
Immunologically, the goal is to reconstruct the immune barrier by increasing the number of CD4 blood cells as much as possible, and by supporting them in their effectiveness.
These objectives can be fulfilled by using a series of well set criteria in administrating antiretroviral drugs, in order to achieve the biological target and also to determine as few as possible adverse reactions as well as a good adherence to treatment.
Equally important is the social and psychological support derived from close collaboration within the team of infectious diseases doctors and psychologists assisting the infected

patient. It helps develop a multidisciplinary approach, sustained also by cardiologists, nutritionists, obstetricians and any other specialist that any come in contact with the HIV / AIDS patient in his lifetime.

4.2 The social target in addressing the HIV/AIDS adolescent

The social target has two key factors. One is collaboration with the authorities responsible for education, in order to prevent school dropout, a common phenomenon not only among infected patients, but also among all young people in rural areas or with poor material conditions.

The other is the need to raise patients' employability, because in the case of this particular population finding a job is difficult, if not impossible, due to the conditions we have explained earlier in this paper.

In addressing this specific target, the Regional Center in Iaşi works closely with non-government organizations such as the ADV Foundation (Fundația „Alături de voi"). It was founded in March 2002 by Holt International Children's Services with USAID funding, and has taken in all the HIV programs conducted in Romania by Holt since 1992. In 2008, ADV began a program designed to offer HIV positive young people a work place and a steady income.

4.3 The psychological target in addressing the HIV/AIDS adolescent

Regarding the psychological target, we consider two main directions: first of all, information and acceptance, and then cognitive restructuring.

When the patient performs a test to determine the HIV status, even before receiving the results, he is counseled by a psychologist. He is informed about the characteristics of infection, as well as its possible consequences on his life.

Everyone's experience will be different but being diagnosed with HIV can create a raft of emotions including anger, denial, depression, anxiety, shock, and fear of death. Further emotional stress could stem from thoughts about who people should tell, how lifestyle will change and if it will be possible to have children. Some may also experience guilt, viewing their infection as a punishment for their sexual orientation or consumption drugs, or for the worry they may cause to other people and for possibly infecting others. Just as reactions differ, so too will the ways in which people deal with them. There is no standard method of dealing with something as profound as a positive HIV diagnosis and it is the counselor's responsibility to find the proper way to approach each patient.

Counseling can be helpful in order to come to terms with the diagnosis and resulting feelings, and as a precursor to dealing with the virus itself. Discussing the patient's immediate emotional concerns is recommended by the World Health Organization (WHO) as part of post-test counseling. Such steps could enable the patient to more effectively absorb information regarding the consequences of their diagnosis, and they might make better-considered decisions about their next steps including preventing risky behavior and beginning treatment.

It is often considered ineffective to discuss possible clinical procedures with the patient soon after their diagnosis, and that this should generally be postponed until a later time. So, upon receiving a positive result, the patient is first and foremost encouraged to consciously realize that he is infected. He is offered support to gradually accept the situation, and to comply in taking the treatment prescribed to lead a normal life.

In terms of cognitive restructuring, this is achieved by eliminating the so-called "dysfunctional thoughts." Most HIV/AIDS patients suffer from inferiority complexes due to physical appearance. In discussions with them, we often encounter lines like: "I am very weak; people will know that I have AIDS" (the "AIDS-like" syndrome). The impact of physical changes experienced by patients is significant, in emotional terms, generating anxiety, depression and stress. An effective way to eliminate dysfunctional thoughts is by replacing them with compensatory positive thoughts. It is the psychologist's duty to give out the proper information, so that the patient realizes his situation, as well as the importance of his treatment, which will reduce or eliminate any sign of the disease of taken properly.

Disability, weakness, and rejection from people around him can cause low self-esteem in the infected patient. To lead a normal life, he must fight these burdens. Although it is not easy, he must understand and truly believe that he can be and act the same as other, healthier people.

In order to achieve these targets, the efforts of the infectious diseases doctor and the psychologist working with the patient are not enough. Research shows that the environment in which HIV positive patients live, work or receive their treatment has a major impact on the evolution of their self-esteem (McGovern, 2002). Stress is another factor that has a major influence, and it has been shown that it may cause a more rapid disease progression (O'Cleirigh, Ironson, 2007).

5. Conclusions

While recent scientific efforts have resulted in a series of discoveries and advances in understanding and controlling the virus that causes AIDS, this progress has had limited impact on the majority of HIV infected people and populations living in developing countries. The social and economic conditions that nurture the spread of the virus have to be confronted as essential elements in local and global efforts to stem its spread and create effective solutions to halt the epidemic. They must also be considered in supporting and improving the quality of life of the infected people.

The fact that stigma remains in developed countries, where treatment has been widely available for over a decade, indicates that the relationship between HIV treatment and stigma is not straightforward. It is not enough to discover new drugs and high-tech treatments that reduce physical and metabolic symptoms. The social symptoms must also be addressed for a proper management any HIV/AIDS infected person.

The specifics of the adolescent HIV infected population in the Moldova area has been widely discussed throughout this paper. Their opinions have been presented, and a clear picture of the current situation has been described. But that is only the first step, because being aware of a situation is far fro solving it.

If in the past taking care of the HIV infected person was the duty of the infectious diseases doctor and the patient's family, today the idea of a whole team of specialists working together is becoming increasingly popular. The psychologist's role is more clearly defined, as well as the implications of the social worker. And more importantly, a large number of doctors from different fields are becoming more and more involved and open-minded about treating this type of patient.

The mentality of the population in general is also changing. The speed of this change differs from country to country, and in Romania accepting new ideas is not done at a fast pace.

However, people are becoming increasingly more aware of different aspects that involve their everyday safety and this includes correct information about being infected with HIV and developing AIDS.

Even though the F type HIV that is the main cause of infection in our country has, so far, allowed a longer than expected life span, the young infected people have grown up with the knowledge that at any given time they might die. For adolescents, it is difficult to build a life on this kind of foundation that is still unsure and filled with past and current frustrations about discrimination and being different. Growing up with AIDS has not been and is not an easy task. This explains many young people's desire to live their life on a more accelerated rate than post persons do. One of the main characteristics of HIV infected youth is their tendency to fall in love and want to get married early, their acute desire to have children, and enjoy all the positive aspects of life "as soon as possible".

However, the availability of support groups, non-governmental organizations and counselors may make things easier. More so than in the past, HIV infected adolescents are encouraged to express their feelings and concerns and a number of programs are developed to help them.

The most important aspect, though, is education, not only of the HIV positives, but also of the general population, that may or may not be at risk of infection. Constant information, constant exposure, are the most effective ways to actively fight discrimination, rejection, and also the spread of the virus. And this in turn might be the best way to support the already infected adolescents and young people in living with AIDS.

6. Acknowledgments

The authors would like to thank for their collaboration and support: The Regional HIV/AIDS Center Iaşi, The Infectious Diseases Hospital Iaşi, the "Guilliver" Hospice Placement enter and the ADV Foundation.

7. References

Astărăstoae V. & Stoica O. (2000) *Problemele de etică în terapeutica medicală.* În: Terapeutica medicală; sub red. Ungureanu G., Covic M., Ed. Polirom, Iaşi, 573-583

Benea, O. E. & Streinu Cercel A. (2011) *Managementul bolnavului cu infecţie HIV*, IBI Matei Balş Bucureşti

Branden, N. (2001) The *psychology of self-esteem: a revolutionary approach to self-understanding that launched a new era in modern psychology*. San Francisco: Jossey-Bass.

Buzducea, D. (1997) *SIDA – Confluenţe psihosociale.* Ed. Ştiinţă şi Tehnică Bucureşti

Caluschi, M. (2001) *Probleme de psihologie socială.* Ed. Cantes Iaşi

Close, K. (2007) Psychosocial Aspects of HIV/AIDS: Children and Adolescents, HIV Curriculum for the Health Professional

Dorobăţ C. (2007) *Curs de boli infecţioase pentru studenţii facultăţilor de medicină dentară.* Editura Tehnopress, Iaşi, Ediţia a II-a.

Dorobăţ C. & Teodor A. & Teodor D. & Ghibu L. & Bejan C. & Luca V. (2008) Neurological side effects in antiretroviral therapy in HIV infected patients. *Revista Medicală de Chirurgie a Societăţii Medicale Naţionale*, 112, 1, supl.1 : 51.

Florescu, L. & Frăţiman, L. (2000) *Ontogeneza dezvoltării în situaţii de abandon*, Editura Fundaţiei "Andrei Şaguna", Constanţa.

Herek, G. & Capitanio, J. (1997). *AIDS Stigma and Contact With Persons With AIDS : Effects of Direct and Vicarious Contact*. Department of Psychology, University of California at Davis. Published in Journal of Applied Social Psychology, 1997, 27 (1), 1-36

Luca V. & Dorobăţ C. & Gh. Dorobăţ (2004) *Terapia intensivă în bolile infecţioase severe*. Ed. TEHNOPRESS Iaşi.

Manciuc C. & Dorobăţ C. & Filip F. (2010) The Principles of bioethics in the nowadays therapy of hepatitis B and C. *Romanian Journal of Bioethics*, Vol. 8, No. 2, April - June 2010

Manciuc C. & Largu A. & Nicolau C. & Stoica D. & Nicolau C. & Dorobăţ C. (2009) Aderenta si complianta la terapia antiretrovirala a tinerilor infectati HIV este in legatura cu tabagismul cronic ?. *Proceeding of Zilele Ştiinţifice ale Institutului Naţional de Boli Infecţioase „Prof. Dr. Matei Balş"*, Bucureşti, October 2009.

Manciuc C. & Largu A. & Nicolau C. & Stoica D. & Prisecaru L. J. & Dorobăţ C. (2009) Eul personal in raport cu relatiile socio-medicale ale pacientilor infectati Hiv. *Proceeding of Zilele Ştiinţifice ale Institutului Naţional de Boli Infecţioase „Prof. Dr. Matei Balş"*, Bucureşti, October 2009

Manciuc C. & Nicolau C. & Vâţă A. & Prisăcaru L. J. & Matei D. & Boghian A. & Largu A. & Dorobăţ C. (2010) Mother to child HIV transmission in the North-East of Romania. Therapeutics, Pharmacology and Clinical Toxicology, Vol XIV, Number 2, June 2010, Pages 100-102, ISSN 1583-0012

Manciuc C. & Nicolau C. & Prisacaru J. L. & Dorobăţ C. (2010) Palliative care in AIDS cases. *Therapeutics, Pharmacology and Clinical Toxicology*. Vol XIV, Number 4, December 2010, pages 300-301, ISSN 1583-0012

McGovern, J. & Guida, F. & Corey, P. (2002) *Improved health and self-esteem among patients with AIDS in a therapeutic community nursing program.*

Mitrofan, I. & Ciupercă, C. (1998) *Incursiune în psihosociologia şi psihosexologia familiei*, Editura Mihaela Press, Bucureşti.

Munteanu, A. (1998) *Psihologia copilului şi adolescentului*, Editura Augusta, Timişoara.

Mruk, C. (2006) *Self-Esteem research, theory, and practice: Toward a positive psychology of self-esteem* (3rd ed.). New York: Springer.

O'Cleirigh, C. & Ironson, G. (2007) *Stress, Emotional Factors Can Affect Progression Of HIV/AIDS*, USA Today

O'Malley, P. M. & Bachman, J. G. (1983) *Self-esteem changes and stability between ages 13 and 23*. Developmental Psychology, 19, 257-268

Parker, Richard G. & Aggleton, P (2002). *HIV/AIDS-related stigma and discrimination: A conceptual framework and an agenda for action*; Horizons Program

Petrea, S. (1997) *SIDA – Trecerea oprită*, Ed. All Bucureşti.

Rodewalt, F. & Tragakis, M. W. (2003) *Self-esteem and self-regulation: Toward optimal studies of self-esteem*. Psychological Inquiry, 14(1), 66–70.

Usaci, Doina (2003) *Imunodeficiența psihoafectivă și comportamentală în raport cu HIV/SIDA*, Editura Polirom, Iași.

Wigfield, A. & Eccles, J. (1994) *Children's competence beliefs, achievement values, and general self-esteem change across elementary and middle school*, In: Journal of Early Adolescence, Vol. 14, No. 2, 107-138.

http://www.avert.org

7

Concept of the Voluntariness in Kidney Transplantation from the Position of Donors and Recipients

Omur Elcioglu[1] and Seyyare Duman[2]
[1]*Eskisehir Osmangazi University Faculty of Medicine Department of History of Medicine and Ethics, Eskisehir,*
[2]*Anadolu University Faculty of Education Department of German Language Education, Eskisehir,*
Turkey

1. Introduction

Organ and tissue transplantation is always a procedure that involves two people, i.e. the donor and the recipient. A patient suffering from chronic renal failure primarily needs a kidney donation and transplantation. The studies and surveys about organ donation demonstrate that the number of organs donated fails to meet the need for organs. Given the studies about organ and tissue transplants, we note that organ donations from related or unrelated living donors have become more widespread due to increasing need for organs. (Lennerling & Nyberg, 2004; Kim et al, 2006, Donelly et al, 1999, Mousavi, 2006, Al-Khader, 2005).

Unfortunately, these sources have so far been unable to keep up with the demand. As a result, there is a large and staidly increasing number of potential recipients awaiting transplantation, some of who dies before an organ is found.

It is widely accepted that the optimal donor for a patient suffering from end-stage renal disease is an adult first-degree relative. However, there is an increasing global-wide tendency to use living donors who have an emotional but not genetic relation with the patient, and this tendency has been supported in the world.(Adorno, 2001, Wilkinson,2007, Chaudry et al, 2007)

The recipient lists and kidney transplantations show that 15% of recipients in waiting lists receive kidneys from their spouses. The success of kidney transplantations with organs received from unrelated donors resulted in the emergence of two donor categories:

1. Donors that have an emotional relationship with the recipient
2. Volunteers that the recipient does not know at all

Although these two categories are different from each other, it is possible to combine them under the concept of altruism. (Spital, 2005)

The life of a single person is valuable because it has a real specific value. As argued by R. Dworkin, religious and non-religious people may compromise on the fact that human life is sacred and hence has a real specific value. However, there is no compromise on why it is sacred. Human life has a specific value in its own rights. This real value emerges when individuals pay attention to the benefit of their own lives in general.

Transplantation is not possible if there is no organ for transplant. There may be transplants from living donors and dead donors. At this point, there is need to distinguish between "non-directed donation", organ donated by a living donor to any recipient waiting an organ from a cadaver donor, and "directed donation", organ donated by a living donor to a designated recipient. In both types, voluntariness constitutes the basis of donation, and altruistic approach is adopted (Matas et al, 2000). Free and informed choice is an oft-acknowledged ethical basis for living kidney donation. Including parental living kidney donation.

The small number of empirical studies of voluntariness among living donor may be function of elusive nature of ideal voluntariness in a population that can be accepted as medical risk for the benefit of others. Recruitment of living donors represents medical and ethical responsibility. Their motives are often complex. Categories of motives and factors causing concern were taken from the literature and were identified from a various in-dept interview. The purpose of this study is to find out the values and problems used to evaluate the concept of voluntariness from the position of donor and recipient in kidney transplantation. We conducted in-dept, face-to-face interviews with donors and recipients. The interviews lasted for a median of 30(range20-40) minutes. We analyzed the interview transcripts with discourse analysis method used in functional pragmatics. Content analysis is a research technique targeted at systematic and quantitative definitions. Content analysis is related with not only linguistics but also other fields of science based on interpretation.

2. Voluntariness

2.1 The concept of voluntariness

Voluntariness is deciding to do something and doing it willingly in accordance with a purpose, on one's own freewill, without expectation of a reward. In voluntariness, it is not an obligation or pressure that causes an actor to take action. At the basis of voluntariness lies respect for autonomy. (Oğuz et al, 2005)

Donation and donor are words with a strict and extended meaning strictly used, donation means the act of giving or the substance of the gift: the donor is one who gives. The donor is necessarily alive, the moral agent: the one whose decision and act of will make gift. (Dunstan,1997).

Voluntariness is one of the main preconditions for receiving a valid informed consent. The concept of voluntariness involves being autonomous and free from oppressive factors. Some people define voluntariness with the existence of sufficient knowledge and absence of psychological pressure and external constraints. Given these general definitions, voluntariness means a person's, be it male or female, acting willingly without the control of any other factor. However, there are some situations that restrict voluntariness, e.g. physical or psychological diseases and addiction. (Beauchamp & Childress, 1994)

2.2 Voluntariness in terms of ethics

As mentioned above, voluntariness is one of the main components of informed consent. Undoubtedly, for the particular case of organ transplantation, voluntariness constitutes an ethical concern for any operation on both donors and recipients.

As highlighted by J. Harris, the most significant aspect of respect for human beings is the respect for "the desire to live", and all other desires and their well-being depend on respect for this primary desire (Harris, 1998).

When dealing with the issue of voluntariness, it is required to acknowledge that a voluntary person is someone defined by law and holds the authority to give informed consent.

In the context of informed consent, voluntariness may be defined as a patient's making a decision freely without any pressure about healthcare they receive, in accordance with patient rights. In voluntariness, in addition to the focus on being free of values, it is also required to underline the need for skillful management and elimination of oppressive factors. (Ananda, 2005, Jonsen et al, 2006).

Human beings are creatures that value their own life. Respect for human beings requires two main components: firstly paying attention to the well-being of others, and secondly respecting the desires of others. People working in the health sector acknowledge that their first duty is always to observe the benefit of patients optimally, and argue that this approach does not contradict with respect for human. Well-being is not used in this context as a technical term. The concept here refers to its ordinary meaning, i.e. being good and living under good conditions. The word thus covers happiness, health and good life standards. Paternalism is interference into others' life for their well-being against their will and thoughts. The motto of paternalism is "don't do that, it's not good for you". Moralism is interference into others' life in order to protect their morality. The motto of a moralist is "don't do that, it is sinful". Both paternalism and moralism pay attention to other people's well-being sincerely. Both approaches see people as incompetent, and disregard their control over their own life.

The principle of respect for autonomy underlines the need to inform patients about medical interventions. Today, this approach is widely adopted in bioethical discussions. However, there may be cases where a physician adopts a paternalistic approach for the sake of individuals in line with desires and choices of donors and recipients. Here it is required to make a distinction between strong and weak paternalism. Both types of the paternalistic approach are based on the principle of being helpful.

In weak paternalism, the physician protects the patient against third persons if the patient is incompetent or hesitates about voluntariness. This may be exemplified in the case of protecting potential donors who do not have the competency or authority to give consent for organ and tissue transplant. Contrary to weak paternalism, in strong paternalism, the authority of a person may be violated for the sake of another person. This type of paternalistic approach is unacceptable in terms of medical ethics. With regard to kidney transplantation, the common approach since the first transplantations has been to consider the well-being of recipient more important than the risks that donors may suffer from. However, it is of great importance and priority to establish a balance between gains of recipients and risks of donors (Gutman & Lung, 1999).

The cases where organ donations of living donors are rejected are sometimes referred to as passive paternalism. If physicians have doubts about competency or voluntariness of a potential donor, they may not pay attention to desires and expectations of the recipient (Gutmann & Land, 1999).

Respect for others' will is the most important indicator of recognizing that their life is valuable. Each life has a unique value, and this value is determined by an individual's choices about her/his life (Harris, 1998).

2.2.1 Competency and voluntariness

In organ and tissue transplant, informed consent is required from the donor. To give a valid informed consent, the donor must be competent to donate. Medical practitioners are required to clarify whether a potential donor is competent and voluntary. If there are doubts, weak paternalism may be applied despite expectations and desires of the recipient. Physicians are obliged to complete the informed consent process thoroughly and receive the consent. That is why there is need for a detailed investigation about the organ donation decision of a donor. The most frequent case in kidney transplant from a living donor is that a family member comes to a transplantation center to volunteer for donation. A recent Scandinavian report shows that donors start the process in 77% of the cases, and recipients request the donation in 13% of the cases. However, it should be taken into consideration that the changing conditions and acceptable donor-recipient relationship definitions may change this dynamics. (Lennerling et al, 2004)

Transplantation centers are required to develop protocols to evaluate potential donors. (Sterner et al,2006) The European Union decision of 1999 also suggests that organs and tissues may not be received from donors who are not competent to give consent.

An informed consent is valid only if the donor is informed thoroughly and makes a decision without any pressure or force. It should be kept in mind that voluntariness is not a presumption or an easy choice.

Voluntariness may be influenced by such internal factors as constrained choice, pain, emotional and psychological problems due to nature of illness as well as external factors such as force, pressure or manipulation from medical team and family members. (Beauchamp & Childress, 1994, Etchells et al, 1996) With regard to treatment, the medical team should support appropriateness of the decision by providing information about possibilities that may affect the decision and by encouraging potential donors to ask questions. The information provided should be free of biases.

Donors and recipients should be given written information about transplantation in the first meeting.(Lennerling & Nyberg, 2004)The information for potential donors should be given separately from general information about transplantation .The language should be easy to understand for most people and rather informal. To catch the reader's interest use illustrations, colour and wide line space. Patients must have a written copy of this information and read it whenever required. The information should be fully understandable for the recipient to be informed about risks and consequences of donation and for the donor to be informed about advantages. However, the evidence about current practices show not all potential donors are provided with reliable information in written form.

2.2.2 Effects on voluntariness

There are some categories of effects that influence voluntariness. Many effects are opposable. Some are pleasing, so they are acceptable. The effects of "effects" on people may vary stunningly. For instance, love, threats, education, lies, manipulative suggestions and emotional affections. It is required to analyze three main categories of effects. These categories may be listed as pressure, persuasion and manipulation (Beauchamp & Childress, 1994). Pressure: Pressure is a limitation imposed upon a person deliberately through physical constraints or conciliation to keep them under control. The emergence of pressure is dependent upon subjective responses as well as the existence of targeted purposes. The subjective obedience reaction to a threat cannot be defined as pressure. Pressure requires a real, believable and intended threat that drives a person to an unwanted action and forces her/his autonomy out of self-control. Threat: Threat is to force someone to do something or to put someone under force by constraining their freedom. Threat principally requires a real, reliable, intended and willful orientation. Some threats may force almost all believers. Persuasion: Persuasion is to lead someone to do an action by making them believe in it. Related to this definition, Loren Roth and Paul Appelbaum suggest the concept of "strong persuasion", which differs only with regard to the degree of persuasion. Manipulation: Manipulation refers to various forms of influencing, e.g. distortion, exaggeration or omission of information in order to produce desired changes in behaviors of the addressee of this information. (Beauchamp & Childress, 1994, Etchells et al, 1996)

Manipulation is neither persuasion nor a forceful act. A person willing to control the process of an event may act according to her/his own will. There are different forms of manipulation regarding decision making. Many forms of manipulation on information hinder autonomous decision making. For instance, deception leads people to believe in wrong things, or hiding or exaggerating information impede people from making autonomous choices. Manipulation may appear in prejudged cases. In such a case, the most useful strategy is to review the information with the patient's own words. If the patient accepts a treatment because of its potential benefits, she/he should be open to possible risks. However, this is not a manipulative situation.

2.2.3 Voluntariness is important

Freedom entered as a ready-made concept into many moral doctrines. Freedom is a mystical concept that may be acquired intuitively. Uninformed freedom is not possible as freedom also means choosing the optimal option among certain limitations. Inasmuch as altruistic acts are not prescribed by rules, these acts are considered positive and are widely believed to be conducted for benevolence purposes.

If an individual doing a favor conducts this act with the assumption that others will know it and thus she/he will take credits, this is not an ethical act. If a volunteer makes a donation to be praised by others, this act would certainly lose its benevolent value. E. Fromm says that only a person who self-devotes herself.himself may be wealthy. In his *Ethics*, Aristotle writes to Nicomachus that the most terrifying thing is death because it is the final end, and that for a dead person nothing seems good or bad; (Denise et al, 2005) An individual may think about her/his acts in a detailed way. After this thorough thinking process, if the individual is willing to donate an organ, she/he will express this willingness. Voluntariness is a characteristic of a generous person and would probably lead to gratitude to him or her. However, a prospective recipient should not be forced to expect favor from a beloved person.

3. What is altruism?

Altruism suggests that the purpose of a moral act is to ensure the well-being of others. Produced from the word *alter* (the other) in Latin, the term altruism was first used by A. Comte in the 19th century, and has since gained a meaning that is opposite to egoism. (Monroe, 1998)

Altruism is the ethical approach upholding love for humans and the humanity without consideration of self-interest, and self-devotion to the welfare of others and society, underlining benevolence, goodwill, tolerance and helpfulness, and adopting the formula of 'living for others' Altruism is the doctrine suggesting that individuals should dedicate themselves to the needs and benefits of others without seeking any self-interest, as opposed to selfishness and individualism. Further reading shows that this concept was defined by the French philosopher A. Comte as loving another person for the sake of that person whereas utilitarianism is to love another person for the sake of the actor herself/himself. Ethical egoism, based on self-interest, asserts that self-interests would be protected only in an organized and stable society and that ethical rules are required to establish such a social order and that it is for the sake of us to preserve an ethical order. Hence, ethical egoism links ethics to self-interest. Opposed to ethical egoism, altruism says that any moral explanation cannot be reduced to self-love and that the precondition for morality is to show interest and goodwill to other people just for their own value, highlighting helpfulness without expectation of any return and sacrifice of self-interests for the well being of others. (Cevizci, 2002) Altruism may be the result of the feeling of responsibility for human beings and the society as well as the desire to improve and purify morally by coping with selfishness and selfish desires.

3.1 Why is altruism important?

The starting point of the utilitarian doctrines is that human beings by their very nature have selfish needs and tendencies, and that they seek to satisfy these selfish needs and tendencies, bodily and psychic needs and passions and hence reach happiness. According to the utilitarian doctrines, the first attitude of an individual towards others is compatible with selfishness deriving from human nature. Human beings are selfish by their nature, and this selfishness is never completely erased. However, humans are also weak beings of the nature. They do not have sharp teeth or strong claws. Thus, in order to survive as a weak creature, humans have to live with others. In addition to selfish tendencies by nature, they also need to take care of others. This interest in caring others is said either to be inborn or acquired. For instance, Shaftesbury says that we have this interest innately as an altruistic feeling (Ozlem, 2010).

Machiavelli, Hobbes, Bentham and Nietzsche claim that humans take self-interest at the center and that selfishness is both normal and preferable. On the other hand, Rousseau, Hume and Kant treated altruism as a part of human nature. Butler says that human have an innate self-love in addition to the tendency to desire the well-being of others. (Denise et al, 2005)

n discussions about altruism, this concept is commonly defined in terms of giving, sharing, cooperating and helping. Altruism may be defined as the tendency to prefer the welfare of others to our own. We need to mention some critical points when addressing to altruism:

1. An altruistic act should lead to something.
2. The act should be directly linked to the goal.
3. The goal of the act should be to improve the welfare or life quality of another person.
4. If an individual is willing to act for the sake of another person, the fact that the outcome of the said act is negative or that it may lead to negative outcomes in the long term do not reduce the altruistic value of the said act. Numerous evaluations focus on motivation and goodwill of the individual (Monroe, 1998).

3.2 Main components of altruism

Cognitive frame and procedure, religious beliefs and expectations, worldview, empathy and self-perception are the factors that affect altruistic approach. As opposed to emotional meaning that reveals emotional reactions of individual, cognitive meaning is the bare message conveyed by any sentence. Cognitive frame and procedure refers to the act of knowing through intellectual knowledge; the process of the act; the activities such as thinking, understanding and reasoning; and mental behaviors such as symbolization, believing and problem solving. (Cevizci, 2002)

With regard to religious beliefs and expectations, we can say that religion is an institution that is based on individual beliefs and social aspects, is systemized in terms of thought and practice, offers people a way of life and gathers people around a specific worldview. Religion is a way of appraisal and life. Religious evaluation requires profoundness, comprehensiveness and sacredness. Religion is a matter of hearing certain things, believing in them and conducting some voluntary acts according to those beliefs. Studies involving living donors reveal that religious beliefs constitute a strong motivation for kidney donation among both related and unrelated living donors. (Dixon & Abbey, 2000, Dixon & Abbey, 2003).

The donation decisions of donors should definitely be subject to a detailed investigation. The primary purpose of such an investigation is to assure minimal risk for the donor and provide maximal benefit for the recipient. It is also required to determine to which extent religious beliefs play a role in altruistic acts.

Worldview is the whole of an individual's or a group of individuals' beliefs, thoughts and attitudes about humanity, future and so on. The strongest motivation of a donor is "being helpful to others". No matter whether the recipient is related or unrelated, donors believe that donation would increase the respect to them in the society. However, those who accept the help, i.e. recipients, may feel guilty or indebted. They do not want donors to get harmed. Feeling guilty for whatever we do or do not do, whatever we say or do not say is another way of wasting time unnecessarily. It is required to act honestly in accepting our faults and assuming the results of our choices and the responsibility of our faults. This process entails providing thorough information to both donors and recipients. Good education and sufficient social support may be relieving for both parties.

The sources of information for donors about organ donation are as follows (Lennerling et al, 2004):

40% Recipient
65% Physician of recipient
35% Other health staff
55% Booklets about donation
18% Articles
15% Patient-training programmes
14% Other donors
12% Autobiographies, newspapers, television and Internet

It is obvious that the abovementioned parameters have effects on the worldview of an individual. Thus, it is required to consider them carefully in determining whether a donor acts voluntarily or not and in receiving informed consent without any doubt. The most significant aspect of respect to individuals is the respect to their wish to live. Other wishes and uninterrupted well-being are dependent upon showing respect to this primary wish. Empathy may be defined as understanding the behaviors of other people in the context of their conditions and opportunities by putting oneself into their shoes. (Hojat, 2007).

Patients who need kidney donation experience a long and tough process. It has been observed that most of the donors witness this process. For most donors, it would be heart-breaking not to be involved in this process as a donor in their common life with the patient. (Sanner, 2005) Further, if dialyzing becomes an unbearable process and the patient expresses this suffering, the donor tends to apply to a donation center as soon as possible. According to research findings about donation in organ transplantation, women and men express their intention to donate an organ in different ways. For male donors, donation is a very complicated situation that holds many controversial issues. Male donors expect that their respect in the society would increase after donation. On the other hand, for female donors, donation is an award to the recipient. R. Simmons says that the feeling of family unity is dominant among female donors. With regard to traditional family structure, the woman is located at the center and altruistic approach is generally identified with her. (Gutmann & Land, 1999)

3.3 It is important to evaluate altruistic approach

In kidney donation, donor is the person who donates her/his organ. To donate may be defined as giving or presenting a good or right to another person with no thought or expectation of personal gain. Whether the recipient is related or unrelated, living donors sacrifice their benefit for the sake of another person without expecting any return.

Undoubtedly, this situation requires a thorough ethical examination. The studies on living donors reveal three types of donations in terms of altruistic approach:

1. Direct donation to a beloved or related person
2. To a recipient in the waiting list
3. To a designated recipient (Kim et al, 2006)

There should be no pressure on the donor in terms of ethics. As mentioned in the literature, 'personal willingness' may not be the only reason in indirect donations and requires detailed investigation. (Spital, 2005)

As we mentioned earlier, the quality and quantity of donors is not at the required level in kidney transplantation. Kidney transplantation poses a low level of risk when medical and ethical evaluations are completed thoroughly. Donors may gain a psychological advantage because of the act of donating. Donors have frequently reported to have a feeling of emptiness following the nephrectomy. They have also had depression complaints at times. Despite the efforts to inform donors about any possible negative effects on recipients, many donors may not comprehend potential negative results and underestimate the risk. There is need to evaluate life quality through standardized survey forms. Related surveys reveal that the self-respect of donors have strengthened in the long term. The literature provides perfect results concerning kidney transplants with organs received from living donors. The actions of donors may be based on individual autonomy and altruistic approach. Undoubtedly, related with the decision to donate, in addition to the autonomy and competency to make such a decision as stated by Beauchamp and Childress (Beauchamp & Childress, 1994), there is need to inform the donor thoroughly, realizing the current situation, revising the information given and eliminating any deficiencies as highlighted by Appelbaum and Grisso (Lennerling & Nyberg, 2004).

Today the decision to receive kidney from a living donor is based on the principle of self-devotion to a beloved person. The most common reaction to living donors is usually full support from the majority of community. Human beings are creatures that may value their own lives. Through kidney donation, the individual renounces something that is valuable for her/him, but without which she/he can live, and thus provides a new life opportunity to the recipient. The donor acts for the sake of another person. It is required to respect an individual's willingness to be engaged in such an act. Respect for willingness is the most significant component of the idea that other people's life is valuable. Each life has a unique value and this value is determined by individuals' choices to orientate their lives.

3.3.1 Being a voluntary donor

In kidney transplant, only parents and siblings used to be considered as donors initially. However, now the scope of donor group is extended, which gives larger responsibility to health personnel concerning the selection and evaluation of donors.

In transplantation, there should be very low risk for donors, donors should be informed fully, donation should be completely based on the principle of voluntariness, and the success rate for the recipient should be high. Today, it should be assured that donors suffer from minimum psychological and economic burden to the extent possible.

One of the most significant problems in solid organ transplantations is that the waiting period of potential recipients has been extending due to the increase in the number of candidates. Every year, about 7% of prospective recipients waiting for a kidney lose their lives, and long periods of waiting have adverse effects on transplant results. One of the ways to solve problems about waiting is to increase the number of living donors. The early achievements about this were mostly the result of devotion and responsibility. Today there is need for living donors more than ever because of improvements in transplant results and increasing need for transplants.

In order to expect optimal result from transplantation, it is required to transplant a kidney to the patient as soon as possible following the outset of disease. Thus, doctors are required to discuss choices as early as possible with patients of chronic renal disease, and thus enable patients and families to avoid long waiting periods for kidney transplant from potential living donors. Some studies concerning donation deal with effective criteria about this decision under following titles: (Lennerling et al, 2003, Burruoughs et al, 2003, Elcioglu, 2007)

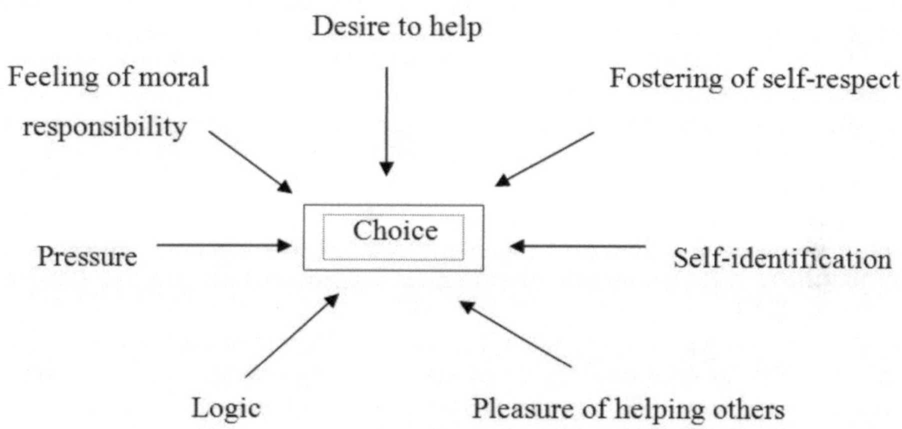

The majority of donors define "willingness to help" as the strongest factor in their decision for kidney donation. The donor is willing to help a close person who is really in need of a kidney. To exemplify, the expressions such as "I have known him since my childhood" or "I believe my life would be more meaningful if I help him" are noteworthy. (Elcioglu, 2007)

Levinas notes that the relationship between subjects is not symmetrical. In this respect, the subject has a holistic responsibility to account for all others, for anything in others and even for their responsibilities. The subject always has more responsibilities than others. Being subjective arouses the expectation that the actor would always take the right step towards the other. No freedom is absolutely comprehensive or limitless. The way to be released from a restriction is to use another restriction as a lever. Every freedom struggle ends with the replacement of a painful and disturbing restriction by another restriction that looks less evil as it has not been seen or tried before. Every freedom celebrated is a release from the most fearful bond. (Bauman, 1998) It may be said that there is a similar relationship between donor and recipient. While released from the restriction of dialysis, the recipient may be welcoming a new life where she/he is restricted by the donor. Or, on the other hand, the donor may have fluctuations in her/his mind while saving the recipient from dialysis and bestowing her/him a new life. The donor may need time to finalize her/his decision to donate.

Many recent studies reveal that the decision-making process of a voluntary donor is based on moral preferences rather than on conscious grounds. The majority of voluntary donors consider their own situation while considering the benefits of a recipient. Donation to a family member is important for potential donors because of their close relations. However, it should be taken into account that moral considerations may hinder donors from being fully aware of risks and benefits. Even just for this purpose, informed consent received from a donor is important in its own right. (Valapour, 2008)

Identification may be defined as a process where empathy takes place. With regard to organ donation, "I would not like to be in her/his place, it is an unbearable situation. If I were in need, she/he would undoubtedly do the same," a donor may say to express her/his feelings. At this point, the principle of bestowing is a respectable act. In ethical terms, an individual must have the right not only to make a decision but also to change her/his mind. The most significant issue is to find the most easily-used method that assures minimum error.

During self-questioning, donors are required to make a rational evaluation. At this point, it is important to make the correct reasoning and present it in an understandable way. If a person chooses to live consciously, there are two possible consequences: First, self-responsibility would acquire a different meaning. Life stops being a burden on her/his shoulders and turns into a decision taken alone. In such a case, the donor has only the order she/he establishes. Secondly, the discipline imposed by the external world becomes self-discipline. This may be defined a lesson learned in life struggle by everybody wishing to achieve maturity.

The potential existence of pressure requires a thorough evaluation. The motivation of donors to donate their kidney also requires a detailed investigation, and there is need to clarify that there is no family pressure on their decision-making process. (Mousavi, 2006, Rudlow et al, 2005)

Influence is also a component of persuasion process. When persuaded, an individual accepts and is influenced by an idea. This is not completely against the nature of voluntariness. However, in some cases, a donor may be forced to act without her/his freewill. In this case, we cannot say that the action is fully autonomous. With regard to kidney donation, there are examples of the abuse of donation in the family. Rejecting to donate may lead to isolation of the individual in the family, or an individual may be forced to donate for a family member she/he does not love. Parents usually do not want to receive an organ from their children. If children's decision to make donation is hidden from parents, donors may give up their decision. Children may be willing to donate for their parents in order not to lose their love. This is a difficult choice where moral responsibility is of priority. When a potential donor is making a decision about kidney donation, written information about organ donation and long-term results of organ donation, high-level care during medical examinations, difficulties of organ transplant from cadavers and long periods of waiting for an organ, support of family and friends, appreciation of donors in the eyes of recipients and all other procedures may be helpful.

As the factors summarized above may motivate a donor, there will unavoidably be some concerns. For instance, medical examinations and tests alone cause stress and anxiety. Going to a medical institution and doing those examinations before the donation may be a painful process for donors. Donors also need care and interest. As they become aware of medical risks, hesitations may increase. Donors should be informed thoroughly about long- and short-term consequences of nephrectomy. It is ideally expected that the surgery does not cause mortality or morbidity on the living donor. In any case, the donor should have the right to make her/his own decision. Conflicts among family members may cause problems in family relations. Although the potential donor is aware that she/he is clinically appropriate for donation, she/he may hesitate to make such a decision. In this case, the recipient should be explained that the donor is not appropriate for transplant. The health team should not distort information in order to exclude a potential donor. Based on the donor's right to confidentiality, it should be mentioned that the donor is not appropriate in general. Honest and open in-family relationship is very important, and potential donors should be encouraged to communicate with family members. (Ross, 2010)

Emotional relations with family and relatives may force individuals to act in a certain way. In case of a disease, family members may feel responsible to donate an organ as if they provide health care or social support. Anxiety is the first reaction given when an individual perceives her/his existence is threatened. The feeling that partially controls the ego of an individual is fear. When the danger reaches at a level to threaten the existence of an individual, anxiety begins to control that person. For a potential donor, what makes donation "anxious" is quality rather than strength of the event. Today's people feel anxiety when they are faced with a threat to their existence. All people have truths that they believe in. Every person has a reason for living whether it be love for success or a person, or love of freedom as in the case of Socrates, or the impetus to listen to inner voices as Joan of Arc did. If this structure of values is subject to an external force, the individual may think her/his existence ends. Given that being accepted and loved is the strongest pressure on people today, anxiety may result from the fear of isolation from society. (May, 2000) Realizing the truth is a function of human wholeness, not of a distinct intelligence. A balanced emotional and moral maturation is required to be sure about voluntariness. The donor's trust in her/his beliefs would strengthen as a result of not abstract principles or others' opinions but her/his own experience.

4. Volunteering: It is not enough to say that "I am voluntary"

Losing one's way in a labyrinth means that the person has lost her/his general perspective about the given situation. We cannot get out of the labyrinth by always repeating the same ideas in mind consistently and then reaching a deadlock every time. We need to be able to put a distance between ourselves and our ideas before revising them. Every movement with an internal aspect may not be an action. If our arm moves up because it is forced by someone else, we just feel this movement but this is not our intentional movement. If we raise our arm on our own will, this movement becomes an action. The difference between the first and second movement is that the former is an action made by us whereas the latter is the product of a movement that we are forced to do. In kidney donation, there is a similar difference between being voluntary and seeming voluntary. What is important is that voluntariness is the product of an action in its own right. For an action to emerge, it should be made by an actor and there should be freewill at the basis of the action. Thus, it is not enough to express voluntariness by words, and a voluntary individual is expected to act in line with the decision to donate her/his organ.

A person may desire to donate her/his kidney. However, for the realization of this desire, it is required that the desire starts guiding behaviors and there is need to concentrate on the selection of ways to be taken. A simple desire does not require such a step. In the expression of voluntariness, it is very important to take required steps rather than just revising ideas about donation. To understand if a person's willpower is strong or weak, we need to find if he/she is determined and prepared to take the steps required to realize the desire and if she/he is still determined despite unexpected obstacles and strenuous efforts required. Bieri mentions that there are two restrictions on will: Firstly, there are limitations posed by possibility or impossibility of existing realities. People may desire to recreate the world; however, this would not be a will. The second factor that restricts willpower is related with the fact that our abilities are restricted; however, we cannot say that an individual desires just whatever she/he is able to do. (Bieri, 2009)

The decision to donate a kidney shows the own intention of a donor. If this intention leads the individual to donate the organ, the donor is required to take an action. In social life, people may feel obliged to do something or prefer to do nothing, going with the flow. In this case, remaining indifferent or doing nothing is also an action. The lack of any sign of voluntariness may also mean that there is an expectation of other donors.

The methods adopted to determine whether a donor is voluntary may be used together. Interviews of health staff with donors and evaluation of survey results would provide detailed information to determine whether a potential donor is really voluntary or not. Organ donation programmes expect to find appropriate well-informed donors even if donors are persuaded, influenced or oppressed. In many cases the feelings of donors may overcome their real intention. There is need to revise and evaluate the donation thoroughly when it is found that donors make such a decision not to lose their job or are persuaded after meeting some family members. (Valopour, 2008) One of the conditions for placing voluntariness on a sound ground is to allow some "time" for potential donors to revise their decision, and thus provide them the chance to renounce the decision to donate an organ. This condition is stipulated within informed consent procedures and has been the strongest principle to determine voluntariness. A person willing to achieve an objective would demand tools and means required to reach that objective. Physicians are required to give importance to the values and objectives of not only patients but also donors. When voluntariness is not expressed clearly and when risks outweigh, there is need to prevent an organ donation. Although experiences about kidney donation have a history of 50 years, certain problems are still up-to-date. Spital asks how we can be sure that a potential donor acts independently and freely, and argues that, in case of profound love and interest, only informed content would not be satisfactory. (Spital, 2000) People may have to benefit from another person's organs or tissues, i.e. organ transplantation, for the sake of the lofty aim of saving human life. However, this act should comply with the principles of seeing human as an aim and saving a life without causing the death of anyone else. In such a case, a donor gives an organ that is very valuable but without which she/he can live in order to assure the recovery of another person, and hence uses her/his ethical right without prejudicing her/his own right to live. Even just the use of this right requires a comprehensive evaluation of voluntariness. A potential donor of kidney has to deal with tiring and painful procedures as well as a surgery, which means a though and undesirable process. However, it should be kept in mind that an individual may demand to donate an organ just because she/he wants to do it. The lack of any effect, in other words, a bare decision to donate an organ, is a proof of altruistic attitude and also an expression of voluntariness.

4.1 Interviews of medical staff with donors – importance of narratives

The medical staff makes interviews with kidney donors in order to find out whether they are really voluntary or not, and the transcriptions of voice recordings of interviews have been evaluated through specific methods. What is narrated at experienced organ transplantation centers constitute significant data for the determination of voluntariness. (Elcioglu, 2007; Lennerling et al, 2004; Kierans, 2005; Pradel et al, 2003)

Not only in medicine but also in nursing, law, history, philosophy, anthropology, sociology and bioethics, narrative knowledge has been increasingly holding a more significant place in the last 20 years. (Charon, 2001) Narratives provide the opportunity to understand the importance of stories. This information provides important findings to reveal mental, symbolic and emotional situation of involved people. Medical ethics seeks solutions to ethical dilemma encountered particularly in medical practices. Narrative knowledge provides the richest data to solve such ethical dilemmas. One of the important sociological thoughts developed to explain the concept of sickness tries to explain the behavior norms that patients adopt, the comments about disease and how the meanings hidden behind these comments influence human actions and behaviors. According to Talcott Parsons, a disease emerges due to physical reasons that are not under control of the individual. Sick people have certain rights due to their sickness, and are exempt from all duties and behaviors they have to undertake when healthy (Giddens, 2008). Patient role is temporary, and sets the condition that a patient has to exert efforts to recover. The approval of disease by an expert assures that people around the individual accept that she/he is sick. The patient is expected to collaborate with medical staff by following advices of the physician.

Experience with patients would be in different forms according to types of disease and patients. People suffering from a temporary disease are expected to recover as soon as possible. However, patient roles would be different in chronic or mortal diseases that require other people's devotion. Stigma may be defined as any physical or social mark that is considered disgraceful. Dialysis treatment is a factor that prevents the patient from being wholly involved in the society. Certain diseases require periodical treatment or care that affects patients' daily life to a considerable extent. Patients may have to rearrange their daily lives and develop new strategies to cope with their current situation if they are required regularly to receive dialysis treatment, get an insulin injection or take a lot of pills. The disease itself may constrain or change self-perception of the patient. This results from others' actual reactions to the disease and how these reactions are perceived and envisaged by the patient. (Giddens, 2008). Interactions that are ordinary for some people may be full of risks and uncertainties for people suffering from chronic renal failure. Even ordinary situations may be perceived in a different way in case of a disease or disability. For instance, a patient receiving dialysis treatment may not want to seem dependent on family members or other people. Family members may not express their affective or protective feelings to the patient appropriately. A newspaper of February 13, 2011 reads as follows: "Y.Ö. (33 years old) asked her grandfather M.Ö. if he would donate his kidney to her. 'My granddaughter asked me if I would give my kidney to her. She did not say anything else. I have not seen a doctor until this age. I am healthy, everything was alright in tests. I gave my kidney to her,' said M.Ö (86 years old)". In traditional family structure, adults are expected to donate for their children or grandchildren. M.Ö. did not escape from donating his kidney to the granddaughter. Narratives help us understand the spiritual value of experiences and clarify our expectations. For many people, it is virtuous to be among donors rather than be among recipients. Human beings have a mind. They narrate life experiences. A life without language is impossible while we live and sustain human relations. We express our feelings and experiences through language in oral or written form. Detailed analysis of the meaning of verbal expressions may help have a full understanding about the said issue. In the context of kidney transplantation, both donors' and recipients' expressions about transplantation also reflect the history of relationship between two parties. Certainly information about individuals should be narrative. Narrativity may be defined as a structuring that connects events in a story to each other in a way that they create a meaningful system. According to this approach, the subject of an ethical action conveys in the narrative her/his information about the meaning of life and ethical values. The narration of each individual is original although what is narrated has a bond with the society in which events occur. Medicine cannot survive without narrative knowledge. In medical practices, narrative knowledge is of great importance in diagnosis, treatment planning and applications. (Charon, 2000) Particularly those working in clinics know how important narration, interpretation and conception based on practical mind are. The aim of narrative ethics is to note individual and historical aspects of an issue before making an ethical judgment about it. Narrations are descriptive as they express human experiences. The described situation is selective because it belongs to the describing person. Further, the expressions of a person need to be binding internally. People provide temporal and spatial information about the situation they narrate. In terms of ethics, time is of particular importance. Each life experience occurs in a period of time. There is need for time for new experiences. In life, fear, anxieties, gratefulness, possible risks or future gains are all dependent on time.

Narratives are the products of the efforts to give meaning to life. Human life is just a series of events, and in order for these events to be meaningful, they should be accounted in a certain order. Narratives contribute to medical ethics through first their content and analysis based on narrative theories. (Adams,2008, Jones,2009) At times, narratives constituted case studies that help us understand the principles and approaches of medical ethics. Further, they were used for suggesting right principles and approaches for a good life. They provide the opportunity to evaluate the events thoroughly as they enable to revise them.

Interviews with donors are based on structured question indexes. They mostly focus on experiences and feelings. The period of interview between medical team member and potential donor is about 1 hour, but may change according to the number of questions and analysis methods used by centers. Interviews are recorded upon receiving permissions required. The most common topics of interviews may be listed as follows:

1. Relationship with the recipient
2. Decision-making process
3. Anxieties and fears about surgical operation
4. Life risks in the long term
5. Gains of the recipient
6. Family members' opinions about donation (Kierans, 2005, Pradel et al,2003).

The content of some narratives provide the opportunity to examine in a detailed way certain topics such as autonomy, respect, telling the truth, consent, being useful, incompetence, negligence of doctors and some specific situations about patient and family members. Whether the interview is made with patients or family members, narratives enable public discussion of an ethical problem. In addition to Mercy's story published by Selzer in 1982, Debbie and Quill cases assumed such functions. In following years, literary discourse analyses were used in medical ethics practices. (Jonas, 1999, Anonimous, 1988, Quill, 1991)

Earlier investigation of attitudes of living kidney donors have been performed retrospect. We saw a need to investigate in depth those motives and feelings that are relevant in potential donors. With a phenomenological approach, interwievs were performed with patients, recipients and potential donors.

The voice records of interviews are transcribed and analyzed. The process is divided into some stages. The evaluation method below was developed by Karlsson in 1993:

1. Transcriptions are read carefully many times.
2. The text is divided into discrete parts. As questions are prepared before the interview, there is already an automatic division.
3. Each part is titled by the researcher.
4. In synthesis, meaning units structured for each interview are used. (desire to help, donation is a humane approach, moral responsibility, external pressures and so on)
5. The general structure of interview is summarized.

As mentioned some papers, the health professionals working with this field have a great responsibility in the task of selection donors. (Lennerling et al, 2003).

Narratives bridge the gap between past and future so that the individual can take action. In this respect, the purpose of phenomenological research is to define past feelings and experiences of participants.

In the history of philosophy, Husserl, Kirkegaard, Heidegger and Sartre contributed to the development of this method. (Monreo, 1996, Lennerling et al, 2004).

The issues dealt with to define altruistic approach from Hume to Trivers have been as follows: family life, group relations, human nature, concept of responsibility, self-perception, empathy, situational factors, costs and expectations. (Monreo, 1996).

Narratives qualify and interpret an event, clarify feelings and thoughts about this event and add meaning to it. These are unique just like the narrating person. They provide starting, middle and end points. This allows presenting an overview about the issue dealt with.

The stories that we think we are living are not necessarily the same as the stories we think we lived when we look back or as the stories that others think we lived. The advantage of looking back is that we (or others) may reevaluate the nature of the narrative that we think we lived and thus redefine whatever we lived.

This is the advantage of looking back: Seeing the importance of an event that emerges after the occurrence of the event.

In kidney transplantation, narratives of donors and recipients are important as they show to which extent we listened to them, we value them, we empathize with them and we give importance to them. Narratives are unavoidably influenced by individuals and their perspectives. As human beings, we have to make choices and live according to these choices. As choices are dependent on moral considerations, they require more detailed evaluation.

Narratives provide an insight into voluntariness for kidney transplantation, involving the periods before and after the decision. Each narrative inherently requires interpretation. Narratives involving donors and recipients connect these two parties to each other, reveal mutual values, and clarify who we are, what we do and what we are responsible for. Thus, it is possible to reevaluate donors and recipients. Through narratives, links and feelings between people become more visible. Sharing experiences may guide other peoples' decisions to be a donor or a recipient.

5. Language and medical language

Language refers to the communication system of human beings. It is a privilege of mankind. The ability to speak is closely connected to the nature, ability to think and structuralism of human beings, which differs us from other creatures. Language is a sign system to express thoughts. Sign refers to any symbol that allows communication between people. It is not possible to isolate language from background and values of the speaker. Language is a mirror of the speaker. It is not possible to say anything about a person who does not speak or who does not do any action. The most concrete indicator of recognizing, meeting, understanding and being understood is using language. (Kayaalp, 2002)

In a society there are distinct groups that have members who are close to each other in terms of vocabulary use, have similar interests, give importance to some concepts not used by others and express certain things in a specific way. The groups in professional associations may be an example. For instance, medical language.

Medical language as the language of the institution of medicine has its own characteristics. It has a complex structure like all other institutional languages. This complexity derives from fields of use as well as styles of language use. The domains where medical language is used are as follows:

1. Language used in classes at medical schools
2. Language used by medical students
3. Language used in congresses, conferences, symposia, etc.
4. Language used in health programmes on TV
5. Language used in magazines and newspapers in writings about health protection
6. Written language used in medical journals
7. Language used by physicians in their conversations with health personnel, i.e. nurses, midwives, caregivers
8. Language used by physicians in their conversations with patients (Duman 2005)

After listing the fields of use of medical language, we need to mention that having a close look at physicians' conversations with patients may be beneficial to help patients to be informed about institutional language and cause physicians to constrain their expectations. Patients do not know medical language. Physicians intentionally try to simplify this language when they are talking to patients. This effort requires the translation of commonly used medical terms into daily language. It is not easy to translate medical language into an understandable daily language. During medical examinations physicians may not always be willing to translate their language into an understandable language because of time limitation. Further, patients with very limited medical knowledge may not understand even if medical terms are fully translated. Further, there are technical tools and machines, and medical procedures conducted through this equipment. Patients may have difficulty in understanding why these technical tools are used. In such a case, patients are faced with a physician who uses medical language and technical terms. This is a very complicated situation.

Patients are generally informed wrongly or incompletely due this complex language use. Thus, it is hard to persuade patients and to create an environment of confidence. Patients have difficulty in understanding that they have to trust physicians and follow their advices. When they tend to go their own way, they put their health and the physician in a difficult position. Further, they are afraid of or anxious about medical interventions due to their limited knowledge. This anxiety and fear naturally influence both patients and their close relations, and cause question marks about treatment. Anxiety and fear may influence psychology of patients and result in psychological problems while there are efforts to restore their bodily health. In such a sensitive situation, the informing process of a donor, who is not a patient but dedication herself/himself for the sake of a patient, requires specific attention.

5.1 Language and gender

Language is a communication tool. It holds many inherent differences. Language may lead to both mutual understanding and conflict. Although we always seem to be speaking the same language, we actually do not always speak the same language. Focusing on why we do not speak the same language would help us reveal the differences. Being aware of differences would help us use language more consciously and accept the differences. This acceptance may contribute to the improvement of communication. We can see language-use differences in conversations between a woman and a man, an educated and an uneducated individual, or a young and an elderly individual.

Studies about language differences between woman and man started to appear first in the US in 1960s, in Germany in 1970s and in Turkey in 1980s. These studies have been involved initially in sociology and then in gender studies, a subfield of sociology. The widely accepted supposition has been that the difference between female and male language is related with social structure. It has been argued that the patriarchal structure and the status of women in society have reflections on language. It has also been considered that language is male dominant and thus language use of women is restricted. Some argued that in settings where women and men are together, male members orientate and control the communication. Thus, language use is based on social and cultural factors. However, in recent years, the reason for language differences has been sought in different fields. Brain studies constitute one of the primary fields. An argument in brain studies says that the differences between female and male brains lead to differences in feelings, language, eyesight, memory and even sense of smell. Öğrek claimed in 1996 that female and male brains are different in terms of chemistry, hormones and physiology. In the face of a problem, while a man uses only one of the lobs, a woman can use both. That is why a man can be either rational or emotional while a woman can be both rational and emotional and thus provide a more balanced solution (Duman, 2009).

5.2 Fear and language

Each individual has fears. Fears emerge in certain situations. These fears are expressed or not. Even though we do not express our fears verbally, our body language shows we feel fear. This is mostly shown by gestures on our face. The first thing that comes to our mind may be what fear is. We may first explain what fear is, how many types of fear there are and under which conditions fear emerges.

Neidinger defines fear as a restrictive feeling of discomfort that emerges when an individual encounters or imagines a threat that she/he may not overcome. Freud notes that fear is the reproduction of a situation lived previously, that warnings about this situation increase, and that fear takes shapes under certain conditions. He also mentions that fear is a reaction to a threatening situation. The reaction reappears when there is feeling of fear. (Neidinger, 2001, Freud, 1926).

In the communication between patient and physician, the fear is related with disease. In addition to fear, patients have hesitation and anxiety, which puts an excessive burden on patients. (Decker, 2005).

At the basis of fear is lack or insufficiency of information about something. One of our basic fears is fear of death. This fear appears when we are sick or when one of our close relations is sick or when we have to separate from someone close to us. This fear may derive from the fact that we have a single existence which is temporary. Furthermore, it may emanate from the threat in our subconscious that death will overcome us.

Even if fears are not expressed verbally in patient-physician relations, physicians are required to try to reduce the fear of patients based on the supposition that patients may always have fears. They should help patients reduce fear to minimum. The mission of a physician is not constrained with mere communicating with patients, developing strategies to sustain communication and treating the disease. Physicians are required to empathize with patients and keep in mind that their explanations should establish trust with patients so that patients can do what is required for treatment and use medicaments prescribed. Further, they should inform patients about medical interventions and applications. In this information process, physicians should be aware that they are not talking to a medical student, and adapt information to patients' educational background and current knowledge about disease. Another significant point is to answer patients' questions clearly and not to limit the information provided to the extent possible. Physicians should consider to which extent limited information would be helpful for the treatment of a patient who is not informed at all, misinformed or is informed on the basis of merely her/his experiences.

In organ donation, communication entails more attention. The physician is in communication with both an individual making a donation and a patient in need of transplantation. The donor is not an individual who has health problems and seeks a remedy for such problems. Physicians should take into consideration that both patients and donors have anxiety and fears in the process of organ donation, and endeavor to alleviate their fear. Fear is mostly the fear of death, and anxiety is related with problems that may occur after organ transplantation. Fears generally increase on the day of transplant. Neidinger lists as follows the fears that may emerge on the day of surgery:

1. Fear about the fact that life is threatened
2. Fear of pain
3. Fear of an unknown person who the organ will be transplanted
4. Fear of post-operation consequences
5. Fear of narcosis
6. Fear of surgical operation
7. Fear of separation from close people.

Undoubtedly, there may be other different forms of fear according to the sensitivity of patients and donors. Which of the abovementioned fears outweigh the others would depend on the environment of patients and donors, difficulty of surgery and many other factors. Media also plays a role in the emergence of fears. When dealing with problems about organ transplantation, media frequently refers to organ transplant abuses. Such programmes unavoidably have negative impacts on both patients and donors just like on any person.

Organ donation is an important decision. It has been observed that individuals who make this decision and donate their organ voluntarily feel discomfort during the waiting process at hospital and have dilemmas after the operation. Further, it has been seen that donors feel fear and optimism and tend to show depressive behaviors. Even if they are voluntary, organ donation does not always evoke positive feelings in donors.

Looking from the perspective of recipients, we see that they may have fears of non-acceptance of the organ or of any possible complications after the surgery. Further, they feel grateful to the donor. If the donor is not a family member, they may be anxious about not knowing the donor. In other words, the feeling of being reborn after the transplantation may be replaced by many negative feelings. Patients may go into depression, have dilemma or even commit suicide (Reichner, 1999).

It is an undeniable fact that it would be unfair to charge physicians with all negative effects and consequences of organ donation. Unfortunately physicians constitute the most criticized party in organ donation. Responsibility cannot be embarked only on the hospital or health team that realizes organ transplantation. Institutions other than hospitals should also assume responsibility about organ donation and attach more importance to this issue. It is required to raise awareness in the society about organ donation and reduce fears and anxieties about it. In this respect, what specifically needs to be highlighted is that organ donation should not only come from the family, and that donation is not an obligation but a voluntary act. To achieve this purpose, it is required to inform members of the society about organ donation. Organ donation does not only mean life saving. Healthy members of the society need to be aware that they or their family members may also need organ donation.

6. Narratives and meanings

The ethics of transplantation can be expressed in certain requirements or duties. The first is medical integrity. Patients and the public must able to trust their doctors not to sacrifice the interest of one to that of another, from whatever motive. The second requirement is scientific validity: the basic biology and technology must be sufficiently assured to offer a probability of beneficial outcome, casa by case. The third is consent, based upon information adequately presented, weighed and understood, and unbought, unforced. Without this the contract isunethical: The tension between self and other is skwed. (Dunstan,1997).

Narratives constitute a tool to provide hope for future in voluntariness research for kidney donation. There is no stronger way than speaking and questioning within the scope of a specific context.

In the society, change should start at the point where anxiety is realized. It is not easy to talk mutually about a specific topic. We, as human beings, stop taking action secretly when we cannot talk to each other and renounce changing things. We become passive and allow others to say us what we have to do. We give up our freedom, and begin existing like objects rather than humans. In human relations we are required to maintain our position as subjects and pay careful attention to determination of voluntariness. (Watterman et al, 2006; Wheatley, 2003)

From this point of reference, we conducted interviews through structured surveys with patients receiving hemodialysis treatment, kidney transplant recipients and voluntary donors. The transcriptions of voice records were evaluated in the context of the below specified themes.

6.1 Dialysis and life

People suffering from renal failure continue their lives thanks to dialysis. However, dialysis treatment causes many problems that influence patients' lives significantly. The effects of dialysis on life were exemplified as follows in interviews:

I *couldn't accept disease. I couldn't do housework. My children suffered a lot. (38 years)*

One of the most important fears caused by a disease is not accepting it. This fear is dependent on the progress of disease or may result from the fear of cease of life. Not being able to take care of children and to do housework is not a fear anymore and shows the patient's information about disease based on her experience. This information shows us how her life style has changed due to the disease.

I had blood pressure problems. I didn't know whether I was on earth or on sky. I couldn't leave the dialysis center. It was just a dream to go somewhere else. (35 years)

Information about patients' experiences reveal side effects of disease and how they influence their lives. Certainly every disease or treatment may have side effects. Patients are required to be informed about these effects. The narrative of this patient does not reveal whether they were informed sufficiently. The patient just mentions the side effects resulting from disease or treatment.

I was a stressful period. I couldn't make friends. I wasn't involved in any social activities. (31 years)

The patient was affected psychologically by the disease. He went into stress. Further, the disease impeded him from making friends and participating in social activities. The reasons may be as follows: a) The disease is at the center of his life, b) The patient does not want to occupy friends with his problems, c) The patients does not want his friends to know that he is sick, d) He is not sure whether his healthy friends may understand him, e) He is so preoccupied with his disease that it is not possible for him to be engaged in a social activity, etc.

I was very afraid of machines. At times I couldn't breathe. I suffered from loneliness. (18 years)

The patient has fears about technical devices. We can assume that the patient was not informed sufficiently about technical procedures. The patients can't breathe probably because of fear. She also suffers from loneliness due to disease, probably when receiving dialysis treatment in the medical center.

It was very difficult in the beginning. All my friends were healthy. I couldn't go anywhere. I was afraid I would look small among my friends. (22 years)

Fear is one of the most important components of disease. This makes it harder to accept the disease. Patients unconsciously tend to compare themselves with healthy friends. The patient above is anxious that his friends may look down on him because of the disease.

Dialysis has been a childhood habit for me. It is just like feeling hungry or thirsty. I have spent many hours in the dialysis center. (23 years)

This patient started receiving dialysis treatment at a very early age. Dialysis is a sort of habit and as vital as water for her. The narratives of the patient show that a life without dialysis has not been possible for her. She has been required to spend a lot of time in the dialysis center to continue her life. The expression of this fact also demonstrates the life struggle of the patient.

Generally dispiritedness. Infirmity, the same bed, the same friends around. Silence and waiting for the hours to pass, just waiting. (28 years)

Continuous dialysis treatment has negative impacts on many patients. Further, the social environment may change due to the disease. Patients commonly make friends with people they meet during treatment. Patients have to wait for hours in dialysis center without talking to anyone. Receiving the same treatment and being with same patients continuously in addition to negative exchanges about disease among patients cause patients to develop negative feelings.

Kidney patients need dialysis to continue their lives. The above patient defines the effects of dialysis on daily life such as long hours of stay at the dialysis center, loneliness, infirmity, long hours spent away from home, scarcity of friends and lack of social life. In brief, dialysis treatment causes many difficulties life.

Donors' narratives about dialysis and life are as follows:

Spending at least twelve hours a week at the dialysis center, excluding travel time and preparation processes. (28 years)

The long period of time required for each dialysis session and the time required arriving to dialysis center undoubtedly cause difficulties. This donor complains that the treatment is repeated every week and takes a lot of time. Close people around patients also suffer from problems caused by these requirements.

Leading a life between short distances. There is no other choice. No traveling. Going on a holiday would be a dream. (31 years)

Dialysis patients cannot organize their lives as they wish because treatment is an ongoing process. Patients may have to spend their life between short distances as they are required to repeat the same treatment every week. There is no other alternative for patients during this obligatory process. This is such a restrictive situation that patients cannot travel or go on a holiday.

We lived with dialysis for long years. We witnessed all problems as a family. Which one shall I tell here? I feel upset whenever I remember. (54 years)

Being dependent on dialysis treatment has negative impacts on family members as well as on patients. The fact that treatment takes long years causes many troubles for patients. Remembering these problems may be painful for sufferers.

If a family member is suffering from a chronic disease, that's the disease of the whole family. You live everything together. There is always someone looking into your eyes, and you sometimes can't look into her eyes. (36 years)

Even though a disease is individual, it affects family members to such an extent that they are involved in the whole treatment process. During the tough treatment process, there are always some people feeling anxiety for the patient. Because of this emotional link between the patient and other family members, the patient may feel discomfort for upsetting the family members because of her disease.

Donors' expressions about dialysis and life are similar to patients'. Family relations may evoke common feelings among family members.

6.2 Dialysis and fears

All our fears are acquired except for the innate fear of heights and falling down. The fears at every moment of our lives emanate from our wish to control the future. Fears related with dialysis are expressed differently in two groups.

Dialysis means lack of sufficient performance in professional life for an employee. I can lose my job at any time. I think this is my greatest fear. (31 years old)

Job is an important component of human life. People may have the anxiety of losing job even when they are healthy. However, anxiety and fear of losing professional performance may increase when they suffer from a chronic disease and require a continuous treatment such as dialysis. This patient also suffers from such a fear.

They take care of me. The life of my family is disrupted. They have to live with my disease. I can see they suffer more than I do. Would they be sick of me one day? (22 years)

Patients are upset when family members always take care of them and their life is disrupted because of the disease. This patient is upset because family members also suffer from the problems caused by the disease. The patient is anxious that family members may be tired of these sufferings.

It is so frightening that my blood is removed from my veins and cleaned. I always think of the insertion of catheters. (37 years)

The cleaning of blood constitutes a great fear for the patient. She has the same fear at each session of dialysis. This means having the same fear continuously. It does not matter that the fear is produced by the patient herself.

The patients receiving dialysis treatment mention have fears of losing job, losing family support and, implicitly, losing their lives.

Are these fears replaced by others after kidney transplant? Does kidney transplant - a gift to life - evoke new fears? Yes, transplantation causes new fears among patients.

I am scared of catching an infection. I have to pay great attention to hygiene after the transplantation. I hope I can be as hygienic as required. Otherwise, everything will be in vain. (23 years)

People usually cannot enjoy the happiness of transplant due to potential complications that may emerge after the transplantation. As it is the case for this patient, they may be afraid of catching an infection. The patient is afraid that all efforts would be in vain if she catches an infection.

I want to think positively about everything. I assumed a great responsibility with this kidney my dad donated. (28 years)

A transplantee is highlighting the need to think positively. Her father gave his kdney to her. She feels not only gratitude but also responsibility and affection to her father. This may put a great burden on her life.

What if my kidney does not function? This is my greatest fear. Then I would have left my mother without a kidney. It will be a pity. (31 years)

The reason behind fear is that the kidney may not function and that the kidney received from mother would be for nothing. In such a case, both the patient and her mother would suffer. The patient is anxious for both herself and her mother.
The fears are mostly related with the rejection of kidney. Return to dialysis treatment is highly undesirable. (Nilsson et al., 2011; Kierans, 2005) Losing an object of love, worsening of bodily health and encountering humiliating situations that injure self-respect may lead to emergence and continuation of affective disorders. Thus, it is required to provide socio-psychological support to patients both suffering from chronic renal failure and undergoing a kidney transplant. (Rios-Martinez et al., 2010; Tong et al., 2011) Chronic renal failure may result in failure to carry out daily activities, weakness, disease symptoms, deterioration of physical well-being and negative effects on life quality. Causing significant problems in family and professional lives, chronic renal failure makes patients, their families and the society pay heavy costs. Donors are anxious that the dialysis patient may have a shorter life due to serious complications. Witnessing patients' life and living the problems together motivate them to donate their organ. (Pascazio et al., 2010)

6.3 Deciding for kidney donation

On one of the days of my peritoneal dialysis, dad said he would donate his kidney to me. "It is enough that you suffered," he said. That was the beginning of my new life.
As it is difficult to find a kidney donor, patients usually get donations from a family member. In the above case, the father says he would donate the kidney as he does not want his child to suffer more. The patient rejoices in this very important decision for her life.
We decided as a family. We read a lot and searched everything we heard and read. On a TV programme, a patient said that he was feeling like a newborn after the transplant. Then my elder brother announced he wanted to donate his kidney.
Families decide on organ donation after they compile positive information about donation. In the above case, the elder brother decides to donate his organ.
My father was always hoping that his kidney would resume functioning. But this did not happen. "Until when will this go on?" my mom asked and said she would donate her kidney to my father.
Mothers and fathers assume a heavy responsibility regarding organ donation. Generally mothers donate their organ. This is an approach usually expected by the mother. Behind mothers' decision lie self-dedication role and fulfillment of social expectations.
Both my elder and I work in a pharmacy. While I was receiving dialysis treatment, my brother was talking to my physician about organ transplantation. After he was informed sufficiently, he said he would donate his kidney to me. We have taken this way together. Now we count the days for the transplant.
This time donor is the elder brother who made this decision after getting adequate information. This is a good example of sharing difficulties.
I am a beloved child of my family. I know that both my parents love me very much. On the first days of my dialysis treatment, my dad said he would donate his kidney to me. He didn't even ask to my mom.
Because of their emotional links, fathers donate an organ to their children with a view to saving their lives. This patient highlights that he is a beloved family member and thus his father decided to give his kidney to him even without asking to the mom.
Family members who witness sufferings of a patient of chronic renal failure feel responsible to solve this problem as healthy individuals. It is a universal fact that parents are motivated to donate an organ for their child. It is acceptable that all family members should be

involved in the decision-making process because this is a problem affecting the whole family. The relationship between spouses is similar to parent-child interaction. Although spouses do not have biological relations, the principles for transplants from living donors should be enhanced to involve spouses (Acıduman & Arda, 2007).

6.4 Potential donors

A willing donor may not be able to give his/her organ. On the other hand, a recipient may wish to receive organ from certain people. Social life and human relations have a highly complex structure. Patients may have to receive organ from a certain donor while there are other potential donors.

My dad wanted to donate his organ. However, he couldn't when medical examination showed he had kidney stones. He was very upset because he couldn't grant a new life to his child. Then I received kidney from my mom. If only we could have found kidney from a cadaver. I wouldn't like to hurt anyone. Are living donors afraid of something?

As it is not always possible to find an organ from cadavers, the kidney is usually received from an appropriate family member. In the above case, the patient says he would have preferred receiving kidney from a cadaver rather than from his mother. He also mentions he does not know what living donors are afraid of.

The patient would have preferred receiving kidney from a cadaver because he did not want anyone to be injured. He also wonders what living donors are afraid of. Has the donor mother revealed her fears? Did the recipient say these because he saw all fears were unnecessary after the transplant?

My dad wanted to donate his kidney. He did. I also have brothers. But I would have preferred receiving kidney from my mom. Mothers have a distinct value.

Although the father is willing to donate his kidney, the patient would prefer receiving kidney from the mother. This is just because of emotional links. As mothers bring us into the world, they are the first person who is expected to help whenever we need.

I received kidney from my mom. I would have preferred receiving from my brothers because they are younger. I sometimes think if it would be better.

The patient received kidney from her mother. Maybe because of the selfishness resulting from disease, the patient wishes to have received kidney from brothers who are younger.

The position of humans is essentially unclear; and none of our acquisitions are permanent. It is normal that such important health problems lead people to think on their lives and possibilities.

My dad will donate kidney to me. My mom will take care of us when we are in the hospital. Dad looks fierce, but I know he isn't. I would like to receive kidney from my dad in any case.

Even though fathers may get tough with children as required by social expectations, they are usually ready to make a sacrifice for the well-being of their children.

Chronic diseases that bring people closer to death influence the lives of both patients and other people sharing their life. Every human action is the product of a subject. Shared experiences constitute the world of human relations. In the family, mothers are firstly expected to donate their organ due to their special relationship with other family members. Secondly, patients may expect their most beloved person to donate.

Sanner states two ways of announcing the donation: 1) immediately, 2) after making the decision. Volunteering process follows a systematic path. The first stage is being aware of the sufferings of the patient, empathizing over time, feeling affection and sometimes feeling pity for their sufferings. This first stage is followed by approaching to organ transplantaton and regarding oneself as a potential donor. Volunteering first requires being informed about the issue and discussing it with people around. At this point, the individual tries to determine her/his responsibility. This is the point where donation decision is announced. Then it is time for medical examinations and tests. This is a process requiring patience. The final stage is to confront with nephrectomy. (Sanner, 2005)

6.5 Relations between donors-recipients and life

Do family relations change after kidney transplantation? Does the donor start following the recipient more closely? Does the recipient feel gratitude to the donor? How do donor-recipient relations continue after kidney transplantation? It is possible to ask many more questions. The replies to these questions underline various topics.

I sometimes ask her if she has ever regretted. I asked it many times. But she always says no. Now my mother is more valuable for me.

Even though donation is a voluntary act and donor is a close family member, the recipient tries to understand if she has regrets by empathizing with her.

I call him more frequently after the donation. I must be respectful to him as he gave me a new life.

The gratefulness to the donor may continue throughout the life.

I always owe a debt of gratitude to him. What if I were in his place? What he did was not a simple thing.

Empathizing with the donor, the patient tries to put himself in the donor's place and thinks that donation is not a simple decision.

I recovered thanks to him. I don't need dialysis anymore. Would every brother do the same thing? I love him very much.

In addition to the feeling of gratitude, the patient develops emotional links with the donor because he saved him from dialysis and recurring problems.

These expressions show that the patient is indebted to the donor and also tries to find out if he has any anxieties about the donation decision.

The following are the narratives of patients still receiving dialysis treatment:

I sometimes jokingly say to my mother that she doesn't have to give her kidney. But I can see that she is worried for me more than I am. Are we closer to each other now?

A patient may develop a closer and more binding relationship with the individual who will bestow a new life on her?

We have always been two parts of a whole. We are happy to be together. We will continue to be happy after the transplant.

Wholeness and happiness are the same before and after the transplant if bonds of love are strong.

Patients with strong family bonds mentioned that they could overcome problems with family support and solidarity. Kierans also emphasizes that family bonds are effective on the solution of problems. (Kierans, 2005)

Given the reality that the donor is losing something and the recipient is gaining something, there is need to inform donors completely about the whole process and not to put any pressure on the donor. The medical team is required to determine the limit of paternalistic approach that impedes altruistic attitude of a donor. (Banasik, 2006)

6.6 Donors in the eyes of recipients

Do donors have distinctive characteristics? Which characteristics make them outstanding?

My mom has always been a courageous woman. She defends herself to the end when she is right. No one can hinder her when she is willing to do something.

Courage, as a significant characteristic, may motivate people to organ donation. Determination is another significant parameter for donation, which is also expressed by this recipient.

She has always been good to me. Her most significant characteristic is that she is always helpful.

Helpfulness is another significant feature of donors.

My mom is self-devoted. She is patient. I know she loves her children more than anything.

Self-devotion and patience mean enduring something. Mothers show this through donating their organ.

She is very patient. She never hurts anyone. There have been many days when she was upset. You know heaven lies under the feet of mothers.

Here the patients links social expectations fostered by religious connotations to the motherhood role. Islam has a great concern and respect for human life and promotes the preservation and prolongation of life. In this respect, organ donation has became acceptable and practice in many Muslim countries (Goldmaki et al, 2005)

She is determined and prideful. She always takes care of her health. She has given me blood many times. She has made me live for years. She is humorous, joyous. She is sometimes furious with me, but always wants my well-being.

A donor who is protective of her health is expected to care for the health of her family member.

The life of each person has a unique, inevitable, obvious, unquestionable reality, which Gasset defines as "fundamental reality". We feel these realities mainly in vital points of our life. Being a donor is one of these points. Organ donation is an attitude far away from selfishness. In the flow of life there is always a way of escape. However, donors refuse to take this way and offer courage, love and help to another person. Organ donation (from a living donor) is related with the idea of doing favor to a beloved person. The majority of the society support organ donors. There is a tendency to encourage voluntariness for organ and tissue transplantation. At this point, the dominant view is that "giving" is a more honorable act than "receiving".

6.7 How do you understand that a person is voluntary?

Asking this question, we expect to catch some clues showing that a person is voluntary.

We can understand from their acts. She cried whenever she looked at me. Physicians should listen very carefully whatever donors say. They don't look at the ground when they are announcing the donation decision.

Physicians are required to listen carefully to determined volunteers because they are aware of the consequences of their decision.

If they go to hospital for examination and tests before we ask them to do so, they have already volunteered for donation.

This respondent regards taking action as an indicator of voluntariness. Thus, going to the hospital for medical examination on their own will shows that the individual is voluntary.

There is need for sincerity.

Sincerity is one of the important preconditions of voluntariness for this patient.

They also see what is going on. When I started receiving dialysis treatment, my dad also came to the hospital for tests. After getting the test results, he said he wanted to donate his kidney. I know he had been anxious for days about what to do if results were negative.

Not only patients are anxious, but also are their family members. Patients personally observe this.

Donors say the following about determination of voluntariness.

A person who escapes or fears can't be voluntary.

One should be able to insist on being voluntary. The first tests did not provide positive results. I insisted on the repetition of tests. This allowed me to donate my kidney. I am happy.

Being determined and insisting are very important. These two factors push donors to take action.

I didn't even ask to my wife. I decided on my own.

Despite family relations, decisions should be made individually and without the influence of anyone else.

My children could also have donated but I discouraged them.

The donor insists on applying his own decision.

Looking into eyes of the patients during the conversation is generally regarded as the most important sign of voluntariness. Not asking the idea of spouse or children, insisting, taking a step ahead are defined as indicators of a voluntary act.

7. Conclusion

In our study; all the respondents were familiar with kidney transplantation and donation before it became on issue for their relative.

The decision was mainly based on emotion. It is important for the health care professionals involved in living-kidney donation to comprehend how potential kidney donors experience this situation mentioned some papers (Linnerling et al, 2003, Al-Khader, 2005)by showing and interest in motives to donate or not to donate it is possible to support the individual decisions.

Motivation is complex because of the subjective feelings. According to our study Altruism and moral duty were often seen. None of our donors mentioned a sense of guilt as a reason to donate but a small number of our donors were lack of motivation Turkey is a secularized country where altruism is likely to be expressed as a nonreligious motive by most people.

Wishing to communicate with other people and feeling concern for another person are ways of getting beyond personal boundaries. Doing a favor for another person is good for human soul. Choosing a nice gift for a beloved person and seeing her/his happiness is also a gift for the person offering it. This happiness emanating from the act of giving and doing a favor goes back to origins of human beings. Where do helpfulness and joy of doing favor come from? Does this mean that human beings are good by nature? (Precht, 2010) Or does it have different meanings? It is possible to multiply the questions and also the replies. Organ donation, in its most widespread definition "offering a new life" is an invaluable act.

Some scholars give equal weight to organ donation and self-sacrifice whereas some others define self-sacrifice as the reason behind organ donation. The reason for organ donation is generally to do a favor for another person. In society, such an action is usually associated with benevolence. Willingness to donate an organ may also be defined as a motivation for a self-devotion act. In a case of self-sacrifice, the individual aims to provide benefit for another person rather than for herself/himself. In this respect, kidney recipients feel indebted to donors. They mention that they do not want to cause any harm on donors, and that both recipient and donor are disappointed in case of the rejection of kidney. (Nilsson et al., 2011; Waterman et al., 2006)

The recipient may be grateful and indebted to the donor by accepting her/his kidney. Donors deserve to feel good with the credits of their generosity. Thus, donors deserve to congratulate themselves by giving something. The donor gains, and the recipient gives. As stated by Derrida, we should not be grateful for a gift. (Vernon, 2010)

In every stage of kidney transplant, the psychological life of both donor and recipient should be observed and any complaints should be taken into consideration. (Buldukoğlu et al., 2005).

While carrying out long-term controls on patients after kidney transplant, medical team is also required to evaluate and follow holistically the life quality of donors. We do not know clearly what happens to donors after transplant. In this respect, it is required to set a national data trace bank in order to follow and support donors. This initiative would be an important proof of the fact that voluntariness is supported conceptually and volunteers are supported holistically.

Strong family relations make it difficult for family members to donate their organ as living donors. Kidney donation from a family member is generally regarded as an ordinary act (Zeiler et al., 2010). Friendship, partnership and family create an environment where we feel joyful and safe. Living in such an environment increases our happiness experiences. Thinking future would steal from present moments. Life flows while we are making plans. It is required to make an all-round evaluation of everyone involved in organ transplant. Organ donation is closely linked with education level of the society. A multidisciplinary approach will protect voluntariness of donors and make recipients stronger. (Jowsey & Schneekloth, 2008)

"Time is a remedy for all pains" This statement may be hurtful for sufferers but it is true to a certain extent. As time passes and people endeavor to be saved from their pains, a light would appear in the darkness of life. The emergence of a kidney donor and the start of procedures would show, as stated by A. Camus, that in the midst of winter, there is an invincible summer.

Kidney recipient reported that might not pursue living donation because they felt guilty and in debted to the donor, did not want to harm or inconvenience the donor, did not want to accept a kidney that a family number might need later, and did not want to disappointed the donor of the kidney failed. Recipients were generally unaware that donors could personally benefit from donating and would rather wait for donor volunteer than ask one directly both donors and recipients though that training on how to make the donation request and education about living donors' motivations for donation and transplant experience could help more renal patients pursue living donation.

The small number of empirical studies of informed consent among living donors may be a function of the elusive nature of ideal informed consent in a population that accepts medical risks for the benefit of others. (Valapour, 2008) One study stands out as the only attempt to develop a score to asses a potential donor's willingness to donate. To identify donors who have difficulty admitting to being unwilling to donate because of societal expectations, Al-Khader developed a measure of "Willingness to donate". (Al-khader, 2005). Sample concept such as moral responsibility, desire to help, increase in self-respect of the donor, pressure from family and logic should be taken into consideration diligently in order to detail the voluntariness and choise of donor. Empirical work in these area is encouraged to inform the ethical analysis of the new living donor protocols.

8. References

Acıduman, A. Arda, B. (2007) A phenomenon at the junction of ethics and law organ and tissue transplantation. Proceeding of Problems of medical ethics and law in organ and tissue transplantation, ISBN, 978-975-420-595-4, Antalya /Turkey, 17-20.October.2007.

Adorno, NB. Schauenburg, H. (2001) It's only love? Some pitfalls in emotionally related organ donation. *J Med Ethics*, 27.pp.162-164.

Al-Khader A A. (2005) A model for scoring and grading willingness of a potential related donor. *J Med Ethics,* 31.pp.338-340.

Ananda, P. (2005) Module two: Informed consent developing world. *Bioethics,* 5.1.pp14-29.

Anonymous. (1998) It's over Debbie. *JAMA,* 259.pp.272.

Beauchamp, T L, Childress, J F. (1994) *Principles of Biomedical Ethics,* (Fourth Ed), ISBN.0-19-508537-X, New York.

Banasik, M. (2006) Living donor transplantation -The real gift of life. Procurement and ethical assessment. *Ann Transplant,* 11.1.pp.4-6.

Barnieh, L. Mc Laughlin K, Manss B J et al. *Nephrol Dial Transplant,* 26.2.pp.732-738.

Bauman, S. (1993) *Postmodern Ethics.* Blackwell Publishing, ISBN.0-631-18693, Australia.

Bieri, P. (2009) *Özgürlük zanaatı* (Das handwork der freiheit) Kitap Yayınevi, ISBN.978-605-105-038-6, Istanbul.

Buldukoglu, K. Kulakac, O. Kecioglu, N et al, (2005) Recipients' perceptions for their transplanted kidneys. *Transplantation,* 80.4.pp.471-476.

Borroughs, T E. Waterman, A D. Hong, B A. (2003) One organ donation, three perspectives: experiences of donors, recipients and third parties with living kidney donation. *Prog Transplant,* 13.2.pp.142-150.

Cevizci, A. (2002) *Felsefe Sözlüğü (Dictionary of Philosophy),* Paradigma Yayınları, ISBN.975-7819-12-3, Istanbul.

Charon, R. (2001) Narrative medicine. A model for empathy, reflection, profession and trust. *JAMA,* 286.pp.1897-1902.

Decker, S A. (2005) Kummunikation zwischen Arzt und Patient bei emotionalen und psychosozialen Themen, Universitat Feriburg: Diss.

Denise, T C. White, N P. Peterfreund, Sp. (2005) *Great traditions in ethics,* Thomson & Warsworth, ISBN, 0-534-62657-2, Canada.

Dixon, D J. Abbey, S E. (2000) Religious altruism and organ donation. *Psychosomatics,* 41.5.pp.407-411.

Dixon, D J. Abbey, S E. (2003) Religious altruism and living donor.*Prog Transplant,* 12.3.pp.169-175.

Duman, S. (2005) *Aile planlaması danışmanlık konuşmaları Kurumsal söylem çözümlemesi (Family Planning Counseling talks: Institutional discourse analysis)* Simurg, ISBN:975-7172-86-3, Istanbul.

Duman, S. (2009) Dilbilim ve biyolojideki kurumlar ışığında kadın ve erkeklerin dil kullanım farklılıklarının nedenleri (Reasons of differences between language use of women and men in the light of linguistic and biological theories) *Proceeding of International interdisciplinary women studies congress,* Sakarya.

Dunstan, G R. (1997). The ethics of organ donation.*British Medical Bulletin,* 53.4. pp.921-939.

Elcioglu, O. (2007) Living donor kidney transplantation: A proposal for model grading and rating in voluntariness. Proceeding of Problems of medical ethics and law in organ and tissue transplantation, ISBN, 978-975-420-595-4, Antalya / Turkey, 17-20.October.2007.

Etchells, E. Sharpe, G. Dykeman, M J et al. (1996) .Bioethics for clinicians: 4. Voluntariness. *CMAJ,* 155.pp.1083-1086.

Freud, S (1926) Hemmung, Symptom und Angst. (09.12.2010). www.psychanalyse.lu

Giddens, A. (2001) *Sociology, Fully revised and updated* (4TH Ed), Blackwell PublishingLtd. ISBN, 0-7456-2310-7, UK.

Golmaki, M M. Niknam, M H. Hedayat, K M. (2005). Transplantation ethics from the Islamic point of view. *Med Sci Monit,* 11.4.pp.105-109.

Guttman, T H, Land, W. (1999) Ethics in living donor organ transplantation. *Langenbeck's Archives of Surgey,* 384.6.pp.515-522.

Harris, J. (1985) .*The value of life.An introduction to medical ethics.* Routledge & Kegan Paul, ISBN, 0-415-01432-9, New York.

Hilhorst, MT. (2005). Directed altruistic living donation: Partial but unfair. *Ethical Theory Moral Pract,* 8.1.pp.197-215.

Hojat, M. (2007). *Empathy in patient care. Antecedent, development, measurement and outcomes.* Springer, ISBN, 13: 978-0-387-33607-7, New York.

Jonsen, A R. Siegler M. Winsdale, W. (2006) .*Clinical Ethics.* (sixth Ed) , Mc Graw-Hill Publishing, ISBN, 0-07-144199-9, USA.

Jonas, A H. (1999). Narrative based medicine, Narrative in medical ethics.*BMJ,* 318.pp.253-256.

Jowsey, S G. Schneekloth, T D. (2008) .Psychosocial factors in living organ donating: Clinical and ethical challenges. *Transplant Prog,* 22.3.pp.192-195.

Kayaalp, I. (2002). *İletişimde insane dili (Human language in communication), Bilge Kültür sanat, ISBN, 975-8509-64-0, Istanbul.*

Kierans, C. Narrating kidney disease: The significance of sensation and time in the employment of patient experience. *Cult Med Psychiatry,* 29.3.pp.341-359.

Kim, S J. Gordon, E J. Powe, N R. (2006). The economics and ethics of kidney transplantation : Perspective in 2006. *Current Opinion in Nephrology in hypertension,* 15.pp.593-598.

Lagenbach, M. Stippel, A. Stippel, D. (2009). Kidney donors' quality of life and subjective evaluation at 2 years after donation. *Transplant Prog*41.6.pp.2512-2514.

Lennerling, A. Forsberg, A. Nyberg, G. (2003). Becoming a living kidney donor. *Transplantation,* 76. 8. pp. 1243-1247.

Lennerling, A. Nyberg, G. (2004). Written information for potential living kidney donors. *Transpl Int;*17. Pp.449-452.

Lennerling, A. Forsberg, A. Meyer, K. (2004). Motives for becoming a living kidney donor. *Nephrol Dial Transplant,* 19.pp.1600-1605.

May, R. (1992). *Man's search for himself.* Delta Corte Press, ISBN, 038-5286171.New York.

Matas, A I. Garvey, C A. Jacobs, C L. (2000) Non-directed donation of kidney from living donors.*N Eng J Med,* 343.pp.433-436.

Monreo, K R. (1996). *The heart of altruism. Perception of a common humanity,* Princeton University Press, ISBN, 0-691-04355-8, Princeton.

Mousavi, S R. (2006). Ethical consideration related to organ transplantation and Islamic law.*Int J Surg,* 4.2.pp.91-93.

Neidinger, L. (2001). Reduction der Psychischen belastung fur den patienten am.Op-Tag. (10.12.2010).

Nilsson, M. Forsberg, A. Backman, L et al. (2011). The perceived threat of the risk for graft and health -related quality of life among organ transplant recipients. *J Clin Nurs, 20.1.2.pp274-282.*

Oguz, N Y. Tepe, H. Buken, NO.et al, (2005). *Biyoetik terimleri sözlügü. (Dictionary of Bioethics),* Meteksan, ISBN, 975-7748-31-1, Ankara.

Ozlem, D. (2010). *Ahlak felsefesi (Ethics),* Say Yayıncılık, ISBN, 978-975-468-901-3, Istanbul.

Pradel, F G. Mullins, C D. Barlett, S T. (2003). Exploring donor's and recipient's attitudes about living donor kidney transplantation. *Prog Transplant,* 13.3.pp.203-210.

Precht, R D. (2010) *Ben kimim ogleyse kac kisiyim (Wer bin ich und wenna ja wie viele)*, Pegasus, ISBN, 978-605-4263-61-5, Istanbul.

Quill, T E. (1991). Death and dignity: a case of individualized decision making.*N Eng J Med, 324, pp.691-694.*

Reichner, C. (1999). Psychische verarbeitung der neirentransplantation.Technische Universitat Berlin. (Diplom.Arbeit).

Rios-Martinez, B P.Huitron-Cervantes G. Rangel-Rodrigez G A, et al (2010) .Personality patterns of kidney donors.*Rev Med İnst Mex Seguro Soc, 48.5.pp.497-502* (Abstract).

Ross, L F. (2010). What the medical excuse teach us about the potential living donor as patient. *American Journal of Transplantation, 10.pp.731-736.*

Rudow, D L. Chariton, M. Sanchez, C et al. (2005) .Kidney and liver donors: a comparison of experiences. *Prog Transplant,* 15.2.pp.185-191.

Sanner, MA. (2005). The donation process of living kidney donors, *Nephrol Dial Transplant,* 20.8.pp.1707-1713.

Spital, A. (1997). Ethical and policy issues in altruistic living and cadaveric organ donation. *Clin Transplant,* 11.2.pp.77-87.

Sterner, K. Zelikovsky, N. Green, C et al. (2006). Psychosocial evaluation of candidates for living related kidney donation. *Pediatr Nephrol,* 21.pp.1357-1363.

Tong, A. Morton, R. Howard, K et al, (2011) .When I had my transplant, I became normal adolescent perspectives on life after kidney transplantation. *Pediatr Transplant. Doi:10.1111./j.1399-3040.2010.01470.x*

Valapour, M. (2008). The live organ donors' consent: is it informed and voluntary? *Transplantation,* 22.pp.196-199.

Vernon, M. (2010) *42 Derin düsünce. Hayat, evren ve digger her şey uzerine. (42 deep though on life, the universe and everything)* Sel yayıncılık, ISBN, 978-975-570-465-4, Istanbul.

Walton-Moss, BJ. Taylor, L. Nolan, MT. (2005). Ethical analysis of living organ donation. *Prog Transplant,* 15.3.pp.303-309.

Watterman, A D. Stanley, S L. Covelli, T et al, (2006). Living donor decision making: recipients' concern and educational needs. *Prog Transplant,* 16.1.pp.17-23.

Wilkinson, T M. (2007). Individual and family decision about organ donation. *Journal of Applied Philosophy,* 24.1.pp.26-40.

8

Tobacco: Actual Ethical-Medical Considerations with Tabaquism

Villalba-Caloca Jaime, Alfaro-Ramos Leticia, Sotres-Vega Avelina, Baltazares-Lipp Matilde, Espinosa-Cruz Ma. de Lourdes and Santibáñez-Salgado José Alfredo
National Institute of Respiratory Diseases, Mexico

1. Introduction

The Native Americans used the tobacco in many religious ceremonies before the discovery of America in 1492 by Christopher Columbus who took it to Europe. In the middle of the XVI Century tobacco smoking spreads into Spain, France and Portugal, and it received its scientific name "Nicotiana Tabacum" in Linneo's classification.

The tobacco was consumed by the highest European nobility, since it was introduced in England by Raleigh and Drake, and in Portugal by Nicot.

Tobacco consumption spread all over Europe, in spite of the opposition of many people that detested its use and gave arguments to penalize this new addiction, nothing avoided the increasing popularity of tobacco.

In 1882 while Robert Koch found the tubercoulous bacillus, Albert Bonsack invented a new device to build up cigarettes. James Duke bought this novel device and the great earnings produced by cigarettes sales, prompted him to give an economical donation to one prestigious University, which in order to honored him, added his name, and since then is known as Duke University.

In 1954 Richard Doll and Bradford Hill published a study showing the relationship between tobacco consumption among British doctors and mortality. This study was determinant to show the relationship between tobacco and mortality.

Tobacco addiction is a serious problem in public health, since its consumption yields many direct and indirect diseases, handicapping many young people in the most productive years of their life.

The use and abuse of this drogue goes against established principles in different international meetings in Bioethics. Although the first established principle is autonomy, that means, a free will about their own existence, it is extremely important that these decisions do not harm a third people, since it is well known the injurious effects of tobacco smoke over passive smokers.

Doctor Ignacio Chavez used to say: "the doctor has a professional duty with the healthy and with the sick, who put all its faith into the doctor". This concept fits in the Benefit principle, which states that the doctor must benefit the healthy and the sick avoiding or prohibiting tobacco consumption.

Regarding the principle of no - maleficency or do not harm, it is clear that many studies have shown the damage produced by tobacco, thus it is a social duty specifically for doctors to precisely inform all the multiple pathologies produced by tobacco.
In terms of justice in health, that means, that everyone receives what it needs, independently of the social-economical level, we must take in account that all the diseases produced by tobacco consumption alters all the social security budgets all over the world. For instance, in the National Institute of Respiratory Diseases in Mexico, tobacco absorbs an important part of its budget, since it is directed to treat diseases such as chronic bronchitis, lung cancer and lung emphysema, as well as breast and bladder cancer. Regarding the cardiovascular system, 165 people die every day in Mexico due to diseases related with tobacco. Thus, it is not fair that many economical and human resources are dedicated to treat avoidable diseases; since they could be used in other pathologies and mostly in research.
The medical ethics has had an important development in recent years in the daily relationship between the doctor and the patient.
This chapter deals with the ethical act that the specialist doctor must have in front of the different diseases of the respiratory system, that actually are among the leading causes of human morbidity and mortality.

2. Ethics in tobacco industry development

Tobacco production by itself is an activity that generates local to general social damages, from its harvesting to the final consumption. For instance, tobacco workers quality of life was precarious, since they had to live in tobacco plantations and they lacked of elemental amenities; 90% cooked with wood, 57% got pure water for human consumption, 31% lacked of clean water for hand washing, 38% lacked of soap, 23% used river water and 98% did not have a letrinne to defecate. Their working conditions also required agriculture skills in order to learn how to manage and cut tobacco plants, and due to the low income they had to include part or the whole family including two girls for one boy in this job. There were also other risks associated with it, like limited health services access, poor nutrition, analphabetism, monolingual, low income, and lack of basic services. [1]
By the year 1900 there were about 743 cigarettes factories, which are basically owned by few families. Since the 90's and under a monopoly scheme, the tobacco industry is characterized by a duopoly. Market control mechanisms characteristic of tobacco industry has its immediate antecedent in the setting of the price in diverse trade markets and in setting the time for harvesting, creating a real need to produce and to sale, generating anxiety in consumer groups, warranting their own regulatory mechanisms.
In 1997, the Mexican tobacco industry gave up the actionary control to two enterprises that practically control the whole world: Phillip Morris and British American Tobacco, which changed the national industry into a subsidiary of these two global industries. The benefits of this acquisition of the Mexican tobacco industry, went into a established market of consumers which warranties the product sale and the acquisition of a new commerce platform out of the taxation in their countries of origin.

[1] Grupo Interinstitucional sobre Estudios en Tabaco. Información relevante para el control del tabaquismo en México. 2003

Tobacco consumption causes more damage than benefits, in spite of that tobacco and cigarettes have a value and consequently generate a great wealth, this is not reflected in social wealthness, by contrary its consumption only generates richness only to tobacco industry.

The consumption market is projected in the future, since its major offer is focused to young people. The tobacco industry is developing commercialization techniques to recruit young consumers, this is the reason of the marketing spots found in sport events, or evoquing certain style of way of life, calling attention to success, sexuality and wealthy people, among others. There are several trade marks present in the market, that apparently compete among them. What is behind this is the possibility of adquisition depending on the income or relating the money owned in a determined moment, same as the taste of the consumer.

The national and international tobacco industries know that they own a highly productive business, in spite of the harmful to peoples' health, always getting earnings and no losses at all, everything based on the addictive power of nicotine.

It is evident that restrictive politics in tobacco consumption in order to protect smokers and non smokers health, like increasing the tax of cigarettes package price and developing a contraculture of tobacco consumption will reduce the number of smokers that this industry recruits every day.

In 1942 the "Institute against tobacco danger" was funded in the Jena University of Germany where they carried out, with a high level of methodological sophistication and a high epidemiology knowledge, the first controlled study about the relationship between tobacco and lung cancer, in which they concluded that smoking was closely related to the risk of lung cancer.[2] There was a serious worry about the damaging effects of tobacco to the health. Dr. Leonard Conti, who was in charge of military sanity in Germany, funded an agency against the use of alcohol and tobacco, promoting healthy activities among young people. In 1939 tobacco was banned among soldiers, and it was also prohibited in the streets, during festivals, etc. Smoking was also forbidden to teachers and for people under 18 years. In 1944 it was forbidden to smoke in public buildings, hospitals, trains and autobuses.[3]

3. Ethics and tobacco control

In 2003 the WHO headed the Worldwide response to the epidemic of Severe Acute Respiratory Syndrome (SARS) that caused thousands of deaths in few months, identifying the causal agent, the epidemiological transmission characteristics and, establishing the control measures.[4]

Let us imagine that the WHO would not had taken these measures, the lack or absence of support by the scientific community, would had posed a huge problem, the free commerce would have occurred without any caution or procedure in order to avoid the spreading of

---

[2] Rose N. The Politics of Life Itself. Biomedicine, power and subjectivity in the twenty first Century. Princeton University Press. 2007. pag. 58.

[3] Poctor R. Racial Hygiene: Medicine under the Nazis. Cambridge, Mass./London; Harvard University Press. 1988. Citado en N. Rose (cita anterior, pag. 58)

[4] Novotny TE, Carlin D. Ethical and legal aspects of global tobacco control. Tob. Control 2005; 14 (Supl. II): ii 26-ii30

the disease. For sure this would have brought conflicts among nations. Fortunately, all the international cooperation and control measures were excellent.

Tobacco is causing an epidemic disease since 500 year ago, and its management has been exaggerated slow causing thousands of deaths. A response based in ethical principles with International collaboration and cooperation among the governments is needed.

Global usage of tobacco and the weight of disease implies a detriment of sovereignty in the countries, since this epidemic goes directly against peoples' health. Public health needs a conscious analysis related to the appearance and reappearance of infectious diseases, the degradation of the environment and bioterrorism.

Tobacco causes diseases in a global perspective. Thus the WHO established the MARCO agreement with around 2000 articles in it, stressing the importance of the inclusion of all the countries in the agreement. The MARCO agreement was signed in May 2003, including México.

In 2030, will have around 10 million deaths by year and 70% will occur in low income countries. These numbers are the origin of International cooperation with very clear ethical and law principles.

4. Global usage

Globalization could be defined in a general sense as conduct of population trough three dimensions: space, time and knowledge.

Spatially, globalization refers to lack of influence in national frontiers, with free movement of articles and persons. In the international commerce it is legal that publicity crosses freely, like internet information and environment pollution. This has economical, political, cultural technological and even health impact, decreasing sovereignty that "depends" on frontiers. This sovereignty effect urges the nations to focus in their frontiers, in health conventions with other governments.[5]

Temporary dimension involves short time to communicate and to travel. This may involve infection diseases or dangerous market products spreading, like tobacco. The globalization redefines the culture, the image and the market demand trough their products and knowledge.

In the case of tobacco, the globalized knowledge forms mental nets around tobacco, that is, tobacco "is synonymous" of modernity, prosperity and occidental values. This creates the image of "global Smoker".

Four companies have 75%of the worldwide market share; Marlboro has 8.4% of worldwide smokers. This success is due to Phillip Morris, an enormous enterprise around the world.

The globalized knowledge is defined as the illegal smuggling by political intervention, anticipating international and government agreements and regulations.

Ethically this globalization about work production, threats nations autonomy and the protection of their citizens. It also violates the principle of no-maleficency due to the use of tobacco which produces potentially deathly diseases, so any tobacco promotion in the commerce has a maleficency effect by itself.

[5] Novotny TE, Carlin D. Ethical and legal aspects of global tobacco control. Tob. Control 2005; 14 (Supl. II): ii 26-ii30

Efforts of transnational tobacco corporations (TTC) distract attention away health issues and they only highlight the economical impact. They emphasize that politics are not directed to children but to adults, which is false. Global usage of tobacco depends on publicity, the usage of image and free commerce. Regulation it is extended trough frontiers with few information and with no contra information. It is clear that justice ethical perspective requires participation of government based on beneficence principle.

The International Court of Human Rights describes standards in order to secure responsibilities and preserve abuses to human rights of private entities. Governments must look for no maleficency from private companies.

Smokers and potential smokers must be very well informed of the risks and damages of smoking. Natural addiction caused by nicotine use and the harm produced in passive smokers must be advised. These dangers and risks are hidden to poor and young people, thus this kind of information is considered to be asymmetric since it avoids a thorough and complete knowledge. This asymmetric information violates justice principle.

The "not safe" advertising for tobacco is not enough for smokers since they have the right to know more about the risks and dangers that tobacco causes in his body. [6]

5. Mexico's scenario

Actually more people die in the world by tobacco consumption than any other risk factor. At least 20 causes of death and disability have been identified (Table I); these diseases are preventable. This tobacco epidemic has been described in four phases depending on the behavior of some causes called as sentinel, like lung cancer. The first two phases show a high tendency in prevalence of smokers; the third describes a plateau and the last one are related to the countries, after going in the first steps has diminished and maintained this tendency.[7] Countries like US and most in Europe are in levels III and IV. Developing countries, like Mexico are in the group I and II.[8]

The nocive effects over the health due to tobacco consumption or tobacco fumes exposition are manifested in the mid or long term, this is the reason of the early morbidity and mortality prevalence most of smokers initiate about 20 years old, morbidity and mortality are clearly identified at the age 35 years. Many neoplasias, cerebrovascular and cardiovascular diseases, as well as many chronic respiratory diseases are the main causes of death. The estimated in deaths atribuible to smoke in Mexico are more than 42 000 in the year 2000 representing 11.6% of all causes of death in people over 35 years. Particularly in respiratory diseases attributable to tobacco, it represents 59% within this group; as well as 39% of neoplasias, 17% of cardiovascular deaths and 15% of cerebrovascular vascular diseases, that could be associated to tobacco consumption.[9] Table 2.

---

[6] Kozlowski LT, Edwards BQ. "Not safe" is not enough: smokers have a right to know more than there is no safe tobacco product. Tob Control 2005 14 (supl II) 113-117.

[7] Corrao MA, Guindon GE, Cokinides V, Sharma N. Building the evidence base for global tobacco control. Bull World Health Orgn, 2000;78(7):884-90.

[8] Grupo Interinstitucional sobre Estudios en Tabaco. Información relevante para el control del tabaquismo en México. 2003 p 12-13.

[9] Grupo Interinstitucional sobre Estudios en Tabaco. Información relevante para el control del tabaquismo en México. 2003 p 12-13.

1 C 00 - C 14	Lipp, mouth and pharynx tumors
2 C 15	Esophageal tumor
3 C 16	Stomach tumor
4 C 18 - C 21	Colon and rectum tumor
5 C 25	Pancreatic tumor
6 C 32	Larynx tumor
7 C 33 - C34	Trachea, bronchial and lung tumors
8 C 53	Cervical uterine tumor
9 C 64 -C 65	Kidney and kidney pelvis tumors
10 C 67	Urinary bladder tumor
11 C 92	Acute mieloyde leukemia
12 I 10 -I 13	Hypertension
13 I 20 - I 25	Cardiac ischemic diseases
14 I 00 - I 09 I 26 - I 51	Other heart diseases
15 I 60 - I 69	Cerebrovascular diseases
16 I 70	Atheroesclerosis
17 I 71	Aortic Aneurism
18 I 72 - I 78	Other circulatory system diseases
19 J 10 - J 18	Pneumonia e Influenzae
20 J 40 - J 43	Bronchitis, emphysema
21 J 44	Other chronic obstructive pulmonary diseases

Source: Interinstitutional Group in Tobacco Studies. Relevant information for tobacco control in Mexico. 2003

Table 1. Atribuible diseases to tobacco consumption and causes of death.Tenth revison of the International Disease Clasification

Expected deaths atribuible to tobacco consumption

Population Year 2000	Neoplasias	Cardio vascular	Cerebro vascular	Respiratory	Total
35	220	297	143	96	756
40	349	461	208	141	1159
45	484	667	310	190	1652
50	739	958	450	262	2410
55	936	1319	635	496	3386
60	1315	1852	794	825	4786
65	1514	1076	295	1865	4817
70	1582	1076	295	1865	4817
75	1482	1244	352	2481	5559
80	980	1146	316	2507	4949
85	897	2350	588	5314	9149
	10499	12291	14321	15476	42588
Deaths 35+	2.9%	3.3%	1.2%	4.2	11.6%
Deaths in causes group	39%	17%	15%	59%4	

Source: Interinstitutional Group in Tobacco Studies. Relevant information for tobacco control in Mexico. 2003

Table 2. Mortality due to tobacco consumption in México,Grouped by five years, 2000

There are about 17 million smokers in Mexico, and nearby 60 000 people die in one year due to diseases related to tobacco. This represents around 165 daily deaths which 38%results from ischemic heart disease, 29% from emphysema, chronic bronchitis and chronic obstructive pulmonary disease, 23% from cerebrovascular disease and 10% from lung, bronchial and tracheal cancer[10].

In 2002, The National Investigation for Addictions found that 23.5% of the Mexican population among 12 and 65 years, is a smoker, 17.4% have smoked importantly and more than half (59.1%) manifested never have smoked, 25.6% was a passive smoker (that means around 17 860 537 persons). On the other hand 1.4%, was identified as a dependant smoker, which represents more than a million requiring specialized attention.[11]

In several studies, tobacco consumption seems to be the initial drug-to-drug consumption (this risk is incremented over 13 times). In Mexico, this has been also documented;

[10] Kuri-Morales PA, González-Roldán JF, Hoy MJ, Cortés-Ramírez M. Epidemiología del tabaquismo en México. Salud Publica Mex 2006;48 supl I:S91-S98.

[11] Hernández-Ávila M, Rodríguez-Ajenjo CJ, García-Handal KM, Ibáñez-Hernández NA, Martínez-Ruiz MJ. Perspectivas para el control del tabaquismo en México: reflexiones sobre las políticas actuales y acciones futuras. Salud Pública Mex 2007;49 supl 2:S302-S311

addressing that there is a direct relationship among tobacco and alcohol, and drug consumption in teenagers.[12]

Recently the Health Ministry and the Federal Government implemented the National Program against Tobacco (2001- 2006)[13]. This program is present in the whole states of the country and has juridical instruments or elements. In 2002, 130 000 elementary and secondary schools were declared "free of tobacco smoke". In 2007 more than 532 buildings are recognized as "free of tobacco smoke". Also, since 1998 the OFICIAL MEXICAN NORM 168-SSA1-1998 about medical records inscribes the obligation of asking specifically on tobacco consumption. A convention was signed with the Mexican General Medical Association in order to receive specific training for counseling. In the beginning of 2001 there were 36 tobacco clinics, in 2007 there are 336, they give to patients pharmacological treatment and psychological support. [14]

From the year 2000 there have been several federal political, legislative and administrative measures. In 2005 the advertising legend against tobacco should be equivalent to 50% of the contra face of the cigarette box area. Regarding taxes imposition, they were increased 140% in 2007, 150% in 2008 and 160% till now days.

In May 2004 the Mexican government announced the agreement with the tobacco industry in regards of the industry contributions and tobacco control measures to the Seguro Popular de Salud, a program to people without health insurance.[15] Mexico agreed measures to tobacco control; these controls are less restrictive than those in the Framework Convention on Tobacco Control, which Mexico has ratified. Although measures to restrict tobacco consumption are taken, due to the laxitude in tobacco control, in Mexico it is difficult to get strict control, other countries could be discouraged due to Mexico's example.[16].

It has been calculated that in 2008 the cost for medical attention in diseases related to tobacco consumption were around 5,700 millions USD. This estimation is based on the total expense in health and supposes treatment costs related to tobacco represent 10% of the total cost in medical attention.

In the National Institute of Respiratory Diseases (INER), the 2009 cost for lung cancer treatment rised to $ 2,974,638.20 USD, representing nearby 4 - 5% of the Institute's budget. The INER is a public institution, thus the subsidy for patients is nearby 93.11%. Most of the cost (63.28%) corresponds to indirect costs, meaning that drugs and bed-day are part of this indirect cost. From the total direct cost is 36.72%, meaning for this human resources, medicine, laboratory and image studies. The cost by day for lung cancer is around $2,465 USD, been expensive for the majority going into this Institute. Table 3.

---

[12] Medina-Mora ME, Peña-Corona MP, Cravioto P, Villatoro J, Kuri P. Del tabaco al uso de otras drogas: ¿el uso temprano de tabaco aumenta la probabilidad de usar otras drogas? Salud Publica Mex 2002;44 supl 1: S109-S115

[13] Programa Nacional contra las Adicciones. Programa contra el Tabaquismo. Secretaría de Salud/Consejo Nacional contra las Adicciones. México, 2000.

[14] Hernández-Ávila M, Rodríguez-Ajenjo CJ, García-Handal KM, Ibáñez-Hernández NA, Martínez-Ruiz MJ. Perspectivas para el control del tabaquismo en México: reflexiones sobre las políticas actuales y acciones futuras. Salud Publica Mex 2007;49 supl 2:S302-S311

[15] Presidencia de la República Aportará la industria tabacalera 4 millones de pesos para el sistema de salud de México. 2004. www.presidencia.gob.mx/buen/'?contenido=8281&pagina=151(accesed 29 marzo 2011)

[16] Samet J.,Wipfli H, Perez-Padilla R and Yach D. Mexico and the tobacco industry: doing the wrong thing for the right reason? BMJ 2006;332;353-354.

Malignant Tumors 2009.				
Expenses in Medical Services	Expenses in Stage	Expenses in Medicines	Expenses in Materials and Medical Incomes	Total expenses in hospitalized patients by malignant tumor
1,241,697.80	1,422,178.80	217,621.04	93,144.45	2,974,638.20

Source: Based in Information by Biostadistics and Informatic Departments. Cost Unit. National Institute of Respiratory Diseases.

In Mexico, the cigarette consumption has diminished as the price has been increased. [17] Taxes to cigarretes in Mexico are low compared with the international standard. Although there are at least two taxes, one special directed to consumption called 'Impuesto Especial sobre Producción y Servicios' (IEPS) special tax for production and services and the VAT which applies to all services. The IEPS is composed by ad valorem tax which is 160% over the price sold to the minorist. This specific component will be increased step by step: 0.80, 1.20, 1.60 and 2.00 Mexican Pesos per 20 cigarrettes package in 2010, 2011, 2012 y 2013, respectively. This tax does not adjust to inflation. The VAT augmented from 15% to 62.8% of the final price by the end of 2010. Table 4.

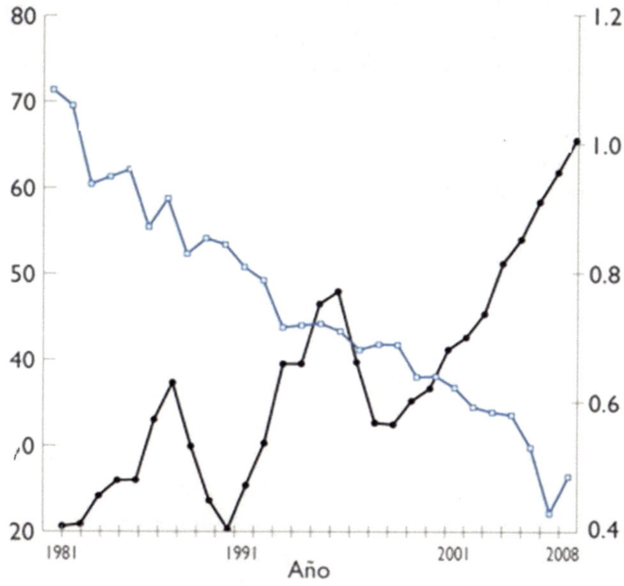

Table 4. Cigarrette consume and real price (1981-2008)

[17] Waters H, Saénz de Miera B, Ross H, Reynales Shigematsu LM. *La economía del tabaco y los impuestos al tabaco en México,* This is part of the informs about economic aspects financed by *Bloomberg Philanthropies y por Bill and Melinda Gates Foundation as parto of Iniciativa Bloomberg to Reduce tobacco consumme.*

6. The new challenge

The free market also fosters the proliferation of industries, such as tobacco, food, and chemicals, which externalize costs to maximize profits, seek to unduly influence research by paying experts and universities, and attempt to control the media and regulatory agencies. The most vulnerable to the cumulative harm of these tactics are the children, the poor, the sick, and the least educated.

The free market can harm health and health care. The corporate obligation to increase profits and ensure a return to shareholders affects public health. Such excesses of capitalism pose formidable challenges to social justice and public health. The recognition of the health risks entailed by corporation-controlled markets has important implications for public policy. Reforms are required to limit the power of corporations.[18]

The governmental task forces encourage further restrictions of tobacco advertising through voluntary self-regulation by the industry, and not by governmental legislative actions. Further research on tobacco advertising in Japan, such as its influence on juvenile smoking and social norms and the effectiveness of voluntary self-regulation, is required to develop appropriate policies on tobacco advertising control.[19]

To keep working in the social and cultural aspects, is essential in order to adequate educational and transformational strategies creating healthier environments implementing new life styles to future generations. Making a difference between well and bad represents one of the threats in education fields, thus a reform in educative curriculum that includes ethics, bioethics and philosophy should be redirectioned.

It is quite clear that there is an increasing tendency of tobacco consumption among women not only in Mexico but also internationally. Advertising and a lack of education regarding tobacco damage are part of the scenario in young people living apparently free but in disorder regarding conducts and happiness perception as they assume it should be understood.

If a government does not respond to necessities of population regarding to health, it is and will be questionable about the capacity to manage even to maintain the social system.[20]

It has been described how enterprises calculate to invest in to those countries where public and government awareness requires exemption related to taxes.[21] The Nuffield Council on Bioethics set out a proposal to capture the best of the libertarian and paternalistic approaches, in what it calls the 'stewardship model'. This model cares for the vulnerable, autonomy and consent. The state most paid for several interventions among them: infectious diseases, obesity, alcohol, tobacco and fluorination of water supplies. The state has a duty to look after the health of everyone, and sometimes that means guiding or restricting people's choices.[22]

---

[18] Brezis M, Wiist WH. Vulnerability of health to market forces. Med Care. 2011 Mar;49(3):232-9.

[19] NippoSone T. Effects of tobacco advertising regulations in various countries Koshu Eisei Zasshi. 1995 Dec;42(12):1017-28.

[20] Moreno García D, Cantú Martínez PC. Documento de trabajo:. Gobierno y tabaco. Centro Universitario para la Prevención de la Drogadicción, Facultad de Salud Pública y Nutrición, Universidad Autónoma de Nuevo León (México), Coordinación General de Investigación, Facultad de Salud Pública y Nutrición, Universidad Autónoma de Nuevo León (México)

[21] Pollock D. Forty years on: a war to recognise and win. How the tobacco industry has survived the revelations on smoking and health. Br Med Bull. 1996 Jan;52(1):174-82.

[22] Calman K. Beyond the 'nanny state': stewardship and public health.Public Health. 2009 Jan;123(1):e6-e10. Epub 2009 Jan 9.

Public health efforts to promote tobacco control are not easily performed. There is a need to interpretation since consumers and policymakers have different points of view. Tobacco industry seems to protect individual rights and that the public health community is trying to eliminate those rights. Reframing public health efforts in accordance with core ethical principles, the public health community can create more positive messages. A public health ethics.

A Framework is proposed to examine how the application of the principles can influence the tobacco control movement. Through the increased use of ethics in tobacco control, the public health community may be better positioned to claim the high road as the protector of the public's interests.

It is well known that tobacco is dangerous for health. Nevertheless is not well identified as causing economical disaster too. Consumers and producers obtain both benefits as immediate pleasure and earnings in terms of market, but they are in a lower level in front of the elevate cost of diseases and deaths caused by tobacco.

The increase of incidence and survival rates, should take consciousness that pulmonary diseases are a huge epidemic, and not only that but being able to have solutions at the health services and also into the governmental level directed to prevent and control them.

The patient with lung cancer is responsible for a defective act, the disease is not influencing to decide the well or bad, this means he is not able to dilucidate or to understand the results of his actions in order to direct his conduct. Family also influence the doctor in order to judge patient attitude and puts him in prison.[23]

7. Conclusion

Lately, the physician-patient relationship has changed, - The doctor used to be seen in a paternalistic view in front of the patient, that means that physician had the first and the last word. The Family often accepted his verdict. The sick person did not have voice neither vote, his role was passive, they only trust in the physician, he used to be at the head of the patient bed.[24]

An Ethical controversy is also present when evaluating a patient for transplantation. Some professionals refuse to transplant if the patient smokes or is obese. For example, tobacco use has been linked to poor graft survival, patient survival, complications, and morbidity, whereas tobacco cessation has been associated with improved patient and graft survival. Over time, transplant professionals increasingly believe that tobacco use should be a relative contraindication to organ allocation. That belief seems to be strengthened after providing education on pertinent evidence linking tobacco use to medical consequences in both the general and the transplanted populations.[25]

---

[23] Ortiz Martínez A, González Martín A, Lorenzo Rubio JL, Hernández Navarro M, Cabrera Cabrera C. El cáncer de pulmón: Algunos aspectos sociales y bioético. Rev Cub Hig Epidemiol. 1996; 34 (3):81-90.

[24] Alfaro Ramos L, Magaña Izquierdo M. Administración de riesgos: Medicina Preventiva para médicos y organizaciones de salud. Rev Nal Enf Resp Mex 2009; 22(2):137-143.

[25] Ehlers SL. Ethical analysis and consideration of health behaviors in organ allocation: focus on tobacco use. Transplant Rev (Orlando). 2008 Jul;22(3):171-7. Epub 2008 Apr 23.

The sick person did not have neither voice nor vote, his role was passive, he trust on person who had the truth, the one having studied to cure, he trust on his experience, and even more if he was the family's doctor, the years knowing each other, doctor was a member of the family. With all these warranties who could be afraid?

To this docility and trust, the galenian corresponded with an exquisite attitude to the patient and his family, acting with intention out of question, everything but the welfare of his patient, even if it was necessary, he paid with part of his personal belongings in order to satisfy his patient needs of health. With this in mind, things would not appear to change.

Social value crisis also affected medical practice. The introduction of marketing also was part of the doctor's tool. The terms now used by medicine professionals are similar to the business people, they talk about management, quality, risk management, etc., also the term patient is substituted by client, satisfaction, that substitute the term used in our country as "grateful patient". The excess of publicity exhibits the merits of the professional ensuring cero risks, this seems to be a generalized conduct in order to that doctors do not seem to be antique. As much as experienced doctor shows, as much as the tariff rises also, there is no space for charity used before to indigents.

What is at least in-patient and his family is the survival instinct and have learn to make his rights value, not allowing to damage his patrimony. Even more, they would not permit to be treated as guinea pig, not to be victims of complicated laboratory exams for simple parasites, they also are not to be in the therapeutic obstination for living few days with poor quality of life. Patients with educational, cultural and over all economic possibilities, look for an advocate, who discovered a new desire fountain

As a medical doctor it is difficult to recognize this picture. On the other hand it is tranquilizing that fortunately must doctors act following the Hipocratic oath with fidelity. These situations have motivated two attitudes: one positive for the patient and one defensive for the doctor. These are the informed consent and the insurance policy against mal praxis. With the informed consent the sick person can decide his opportunity to choose the examinations or treatments, without loosing autonomy.[26] Papers to fill up in augment, attention seems to be tedious but with an explanation gives support and tranquility to both parts. Insurance contributes to tranquility, that means, that is not matter of the great knowledge in science the doctor has, he is human and fallible, he can also be protected from bad intentions.

All seems to be concluded but the patient-doctor relationship is not finished. We have to rescue our image. New generations of pneumologyst need to include into their school curriculum matters regarding humanism, and all signatures by ethics, deontology and bioethics. But not only that, they need to observe and absorb from their professors who have to show their values and virtues as they teach, as they cure, as they accompany.

If government looses credibility by society, the professionals in public health should not be worried about drugs prevention if the trend to global economy is legalize them, their function should be to demand security in health that includes to reinsert ill people into society, with perfect knowledge of what is well or wrong without recruing them, prohibiting and lacking freedom

[26] Alfaro Ramos L, Magaña Izquierdo M. Realidades conceptuales del consentimiento informado para la seguridad del médico y del paciente. Rev Nal Enf Resp Mex 2008; 21(3):213-220.

8. References

Alfaro Ramos L, Magaña Izquierdo M. Realidades conceptuales del consentimiento informado para la seguridad del médico y del paciente. Rev Nal Enf Resp Mex 2008; 21(3):213-220.

Alfaro Ramos L, Magaña Izquierdo M. Administración de riesgos: Medicina Preventiva para médicos y organizaciones de salud. Rev Nal Enf Resp Mex 2009; 22(2):137-143.

Brezis M, Wiist WH. Vulnerability of health to market forces. Med Care. 2011 Mar;49(3):232-9.

Calman K. Beyond the 'nanny state': stewardship and public health.Public Health. 2009 Jan;123(1):e6-e10. Epub 2009 Jan 9.

Corrao MA, Guindon GE, Sharma N, Shokoohi DF [eds.] Tobacco Control Tobacco Control Country Profile, American Cancer Society, Atlanta, GA, 2000.

Ehlers SL. Ethical analysis and consideration of health behaviors in organ allocation: focus on tobacco use. Transplant Rev (Orlando). 2008 Jul;22(3):171-7. Epub 2008 Apr 23.

Grupo Interinstitucional sobre Estudios en Tabaco. Información relevante para el control del tabaquismo en México. 2003

Hernández-Ávila M, Rodríguez-Ajenjo CJ, García-Handal KM, Ibáñez-Hernández NA, Martínez-Ruiz MJ. Perspectivas para el control del tabaquismo en México: reflexiones sobre las políticas actuales y acciones futuras. Salud Publica Mex 2007;49 supl 2:S302-S311

Kozlowski LT, Edwards BQ. "Not safe" is not enough: smokers have a right to know more than there is no safe tobacco product. Tob Control 2005 14 (supl II) 113-117.

Kuri-Morales PA, González-Roldán JF, Hoy MJ, Cortés-Ramírez M. Epidemiología del tabaquismo en México. Salud Publica Mex 2006;48 supl I:S91-S98.

Medina-Mora ME, Peña-Corona MP, Cravioto P, Villatoro J, Kuri P. Del tabaco al uso de otras drogas: ¿el uso temprano de tabaco aumenta la probabilidad de usar otras drogas? Salud Publica Mex 2002;44 supl 1: S109-S115

Moreno García D, Cantú Martínez PC. Documento de trabajo:. Gobierno y tabaco. Centro Universitario para la Prevención de la Drogadicción, Facultad de Salud Pública y Nutrición, Universidad Autónoma de Nuevo León (México) *Coordinación General de Investigación, Facultad de Salud Pública y Nutrición, Universidad Autónoma de Nuevo León (México)

NippoSone T. Effects of tobacco advertising regulations in various countries Koshu Eisei Zasshi. 1995 Dec;42(12):1017-28.

Novotny TE, Carlin D. Ethical and legal aspects of global tobacco control. Tob. Control 2005; 14 (Supl. II): ii 26-ii30

Ortiz Martínez A, González Martín A, Lorenzo Rubio JL, Hernández Navarro M, Cabrera Cabrera C. El cáncer de pulmón: Algunos aspectos sociales y bioético. Rev Cub Hig Epidemiol. 1996; 34 (3):81-90.

Poctor R. *Racial Hygiene: Medicine under the Nazis*. Cambridge, Mass./London; Harvard University Press. 1988. Citado en N. Rose (cita anterior, pag. 58)

Pollock D. Forty years on: a war to recognize and win. How the tobacco industry has survived the revelations on smoking and health. Br Med Bull. 1996 Jan;52(1):174-82.

Programa Nacional contra las Adicciones. Programa contra el Tabaquismo. Secretaría de Salud/Consejo Nacional contra las Adicciones. México, 2000.

Presidencia de la República Aportará la industria tabacalera 4 millones de pesos para el sistema de salud de México. 2004.www.presidencia.gob.mx/buen/'?contenido=8281&pagina=151(accesed 29 marzo 2011)

Rose N. *The Politics of Life Itself. Biomedicine, power and subjectivity in the twenty.first Century* Princeton University Press. 2007. pag 58

Samet J.,Wipfli H, Perez-Padilla R and Yach D. Mexico and the tobacco industry: doing the wrong thing for the right reason? BMJ 2006;332;353-354.

Waters H, Saénz de Miera B, Ross H, Reynales Shigematsu LM. *La economía del tabaco y los impuestos al tabaco en México,* This is part of the informs about economic aspects financed by *Bloomberg Philanthropies y por Bill and Melinda Gates Foundation as parto of Iniciativa Bloomberg to Reduce tobacco consumme.*

9

Screens for Life: *In DNA We Trust*

Evelyne Shuster
Research Ethics and Compliance
Philadelphia Veterans Affairs Medical Center and
Former Lecturer in Ethics, School of Engineers
and Applied Sciences, University of Pennsylvania
United States of America

1. Introduction

Health is today genetic. To be sick is to have been made "defective," a bad "terroir" which produces defective products, made up of genetic errors, DNA misspelling, and so called "disease genes." Prevention, not treatment, is the only option. But it is not that simple. The correlation between "terroir" and products, i.e. between genes and diseases, genotype and phenotype is often not a straightforward causation. Most conditions are linked to multiple gene variations, difficult to interpret. To decipher the human genome is a complicated task, and one that has increasingly become the "stuff" of everyday life of modern adults in the twenty first century.

Scientists have helped the process of "geneticizing" human existence, by announcing, in fanfare, and five years ahead of schedule, the completion in 2000 of the Human Genome Project - the mapping and the sequencing of the human genome. Shortly after, James Watson, the co-discoverer of the DNA structure, and J. Craig Venter, the inventor of the 'shotgun' sequencing strategy used to decode the genome, have their own DNA sequenced, published and publicized in the media. Observers wonder whether the "1,000- Dollar Genome" would be next and genome mapping a "must have" for the not so rich and famous. The Socratic moral imperative "Know Thyself," gains a new meaning, "Know Thy Genes;" unravel who you are at a sub-molecular level.

For-profit genomic companies such as *23&me* and *Navigenics*, have already offered DNA screening to their paying members, and successfully convinced them that there is a near 100% causative effect between gene variations and diseases: genomic screens can help detect and prevent health risks. These direct-to-consumer companies have used a new technology, so called "gene chip" to screen thousands of genes simultaneously and identify mutations that are known to correlate to diseases. A gene variation, for example, may correlate to a marker for a heart condition, and it is argued that the person has a higher chance of developing heart disease and ought to do something to prevent it. The question is, of course, what? Disease causation is complicated, and meaningful prediction based on genomics is at best tentative. For example, 20 genes may correlate to a person height, these genes only explain 3% of height variation between people, or about 1/3 of an inch of the variation in height.

Nowhere in medicine has genetic science been more pervasive than in fertility clinics and prenatal care services. Whereas, in a not so distant past, pregnant patients could only be "screened" for conditions such as Down's syndrome or trisomies, today, they may choose among a variety of genetic conditions that may affect the health of the child-to be. DNA microarray or "gene chips" currently being explored in research settings may allow screening for thousands of genes at once, and once introduced in clinical practice may be requested by prospective parents concerned about the health of their future child. The next step would be to make the whole fetal genome sequencing (WGS) available to the pregnant patient, once free fetal DNA can be easily extracted from maternal blood. The whole fetal genome sequencing could introduce a difference in kind, compared to more traditional screening methods because of the amount of information it produces at once.

Prospective parents want their babies to be healthy and are willing to submit to all kinds of screening tests, inconveniences and burdens for it. Prenatal screening gives them comfort and reassurance that the pregnancy is going well. But a "normal" fetal screen may be inaccurate (false negative) and thus misguiding, and an "abnormal" screen may be misleading (false positive), and even harmful, i.e. putting the pregnancy at harm's way through additional genetic tests. How to manage and use prenatal screens and the amount of genetic information they generate are critical if the goal is to promote rather than prevent the birth of healthy babies. Can a reasonable argument be made in favor of using these new screens in routine prenatal care, to ensure that the benefits outweigh the harm?

One of the most memorable moments in my professional life was when I took issue on these very questions with Israel Nisand, a celebrated and enormously influential French obstetrician-gynecologist. The question was: Are physicians obligated to disclose to their pregnant patients all they know about their fetuses despite serious concerns that patients may use this information to unnecessarily terminate the pregnancy? The debate took place in Monaco, in April 2000, during the International Symposium on *Procreation and the Rights of the Child,* sponsored by AMADE (*Association Mondiale des Amis de l'Enfance, or World Association of Children's Friends),* and UNESCO (*United Nations Educational, Scientific and Cultural Organization*), two internationally known organizations whose mission is to undertake, support and promote all initiatives relevant to the interests and protection of children around the world - UNESCO since its creation in 1949, and AMADE since 1963 when Princess Grace of Monaco founded the organization " whose purpose is to ensure or make ensure the physical, moral and spiritual welfare of children throughout the world without any distinction as to race, sex, nationality or religion and in a spirit of complete independence."

More than 500 people representing about 25 nations were in attendance at the opening session at the Auditorium-Rainier III, which faces the sumptuous palace of Prince Rainier and Princess Grace bordering the vividly colorful, sunny harbor. My intervention at the Plenary Session on *Human Cloning* caused little public debate. The prospect of human cloning is viewed around the world with such repulsion and moral condemnation (as a violation of the right of a child to be born with an "open future," and an assault to human dignity) that the nations of the world seemed to have reached a tacit agreement against its being attempted or carried out. And the UNESCO *Universal* Declaration *on the Human Genome and Human Rights,* has made it clear in its recommendation, Article 11 that "Practices which are contrary to human dignity, such as reproductive cloning of human beings, shall not be permitted." (The difficulties in enforcing the prohibition against human "reproductive" cloning resided elsewhere, in the linkage of human replication cloning -the making of human clones- and research cloning -also called therapeutic cloning- or the making cloned embryos for stem cell research. Most countries have found it scientifically beneficial to do nuclear transfer cloning for research purposes but not reproduction cloning to make a clone child. They wanted to prohibit replication cloning or the making of human clones, and not research cloning.) At any rate, the ensuing round table discussion drifted away from human replication cloning and towards prenatal genetic screening – a practice that has become increasingly more sophisticated and is today being challenged by the deployment of new technological screens, such as the advent of the whole genome sequencing. To many in the audience, prenatal genetic screening has been associated with eugenics (or selected breeding) of past years. The growth of genetic knowledge has spurred a massive explosion in new screening technologies and the fear has been that this could provide eugenicists the tools they have been looking for to further their program, i.e., to weed out all "defective' or undesirable embryos or those unfit to belong to the "human race."

In the USA, there has been no overarching principle to help decide whether an existing or a new prenatal screen should be routinely offered to patients. Prenatal screening policy has been hampered by ongoing abortion controversy, with the right-to-life position opposing any fetal screening on the basis that it could be used to justify prevention of a birth, and the pro-choice position affirming parental autonomy and favoring parental right to almost any fetal intervention, including unlimited access to information about fetuses. Because of the abortion controversy and to avoid charges of eugenics, prenatal counseling has been, by and large, non-directive, and respectful of parental decisions.

Citing his own practice, Israel Nisand publically defended his decision *not* to inform his pregnant patients of finding he considered inconsequential or inconclusive because of fear that patients may use it to terminate a wanted pregnancy.[1] Findings that indicate , for example, "minor" conditions, such as polydigitalism, clef-palate or lip, short limbs, and conditions that could be corrected at (or soon after) birth, or treatable in time of the screen; findings that reveal anomalous conditions of unknown origin or clinical significance may, for Nisand, be justifiably kept undisclosed to the pregnant patient. According to Nisand, disclosure of such findings may cause more harm than good to the pregnant patient (and her physician), and therefore be irresponsible. It would put physicians in an undesirable position of terminating (unnecessarily) a wanted pregnancy at the request of the pregnant patient who may fear that her fetus may have additional (and more severe) medical problems and physicians cannot guarantee her that it doesn't. Nisand also explained, that "Out of 750, 000 pregnant women, 550, 000 undergo prenatal screening using maternal blood sample - a non invasive medical procedure which entails almost no risk. Ten percent of these women (or 55,000) may show an increased risk in Trisomy and will undergo an invasive procedure such as amniocentesis or chorionic villus sampling (CVS) to confirm or refute screening results. These procedures impose small but potentially significant risks (about 1 to 2%) to both the fetus and the mother. (Noninvasive screening of fetal aneuploidy are also available, such as ultrasound but have limited reliability). This means that, at the very least, a total of 550 fetuses will be aborted, 280 of which will be "true trisomy" and 270 fetuses will be healthy.... (in other words), for one "trisomy" identified, two healthy fetuses are aborted. This is unacceptable to physicians and tragic to patients who want so desperately a baby....(in all), These situations are tragic for those who want a child and of serious concerns to physicians who find no satisfactory pleasure in aborting "healthy" fetuses. Unchecked disclosure of fetal findings undermines the original prenatal screening purpose which is to promote rather than prevent the birth of healthy babies." [1,2]

French philosopher-physician, Georges Canguilhem perceptively noted decades ago, that health, disease, and normality are not properties of the molecules or genes, and thus may not be inferred from molecular or genetic readings.[3] These are the result of the interaction between the entire organism and its environment. And thus, at the molecular or sub-molecular level health, disease, and normalcy have no meaning. This observation may highlight the difficulties in determining the health of a fetus at the genetic (microscopic) level, and to articulate prenatal screening practice and policy on the basis of such a determination.

Though this might explain the reluctance to disclose all that is known about a fetus' genetic make-up, it remains that I couldn't disagree more with Nisand's decision not to disclose to his pregnant patients what he knew about their fetuses. This struck me (and I recall, the entire audience in Monaco, as well) as utterly patronizing to women and ethically unacceptable. To withhold information because of doctors' concerns that their patients may use it to make a decision they do not approve of, is, I was convinced, a violation of a woman's right to autonomy and informed consent. It was, as I argued then, to favor beneficence, i.e. doing good based on the physician's assessment of harm/benefit of information disclosure, at the expense of respect for persons and their rights to make an informed choice and self-determination.

I did not expect Nisand and colleagues to agree, and they didn't. But I stood firm on my position, convinced that patients have the right to be informed of all we know about their fetuses. I vehemently argued that an ethical physician is responsible for carefully explaining risks and benefits of screening and the meaning of the findings, and when satisfied that the patient understood the information provided , the physician should respect the patient's decision, even if in disagreement with it. I made it clear that non disclosure (or withholding) of prenatal information for any reason is ethically unacceptable. It violates the human rights of women, and undermines the fundamental tenets of medical ethics - respect for persons, autonomy and beneficence. Little did I know that Nisand's proposition would deserve serious attention in light of new genetic screens.

2. DNA microarray prenatal screening: Challenges to informed consent

An opportunity to revisit this issue presented itself at the occasion of the 2003 international symposium on *Prenatal Diagnosis*, in Buenos Aires, sponsored by the *American College of Obstetricians and Gynecologists.* The question raised was whether the use of DNA microarray to screen fetuses could undermine the informed consent requirement in the doctor-patient relationships. My position in Monaco was clear: there is no finding, the insignificance of which is such that it warrants non- disclosure: Pregnant patients must be informed of what physicians know about their fetuses. But is this still feasible, practical or meaningful in light of new fetal genetic screens? This was the question I began to raise in Buenos Ares. What goes on here? The question belongs in the present tense because it is by no means settled. This is why[4].

Historically, in the United States, screening practice has been conducted one condition at a time, beginning with the detection of Down syndrome. Women aged 35 years or older were offered amniocentesis to screen for this syndrome. Selection of this cut-off age for screening was an attempt to balance the risk that a baby would be affected by a chromosomal disorder with the risk that spontaneous fetal loss would result from amniocentesis. Presently, prenatal screening includes use of maternal blood to test for α-fetoprotein, human chorionic gonadotropin, and β-unconjugated oestriol. Quad screening also tests for dimeric inhibin A.

The use of a maternal blood sample rather than amniotic fluid led to the recommendation that all pregnant women should be screened for Down's syndrome and neural-tube defects, such as anencephaly and spina bifida. Cost-benefit analysis, together with counseling of patients and informed consent, has been used to decide whether any additional disorders should be screened for. Every decision has been made—one disorder at a time— after a systematic examination of its implications by professional associations (such as the American College of Obstetricians and Gynecologists and the American College of Medical Genetics) that make recommendations for clinical application. These recommendations have been informed by the severity of the disorder and the accuracy of the screening interventions. In 2007, the American College of Obstetricians and Gynecologists recommended that *all* women who present for prenatal care before 20 weeks of gestation be offered screening and invasive diagnostic testing for aneuploidy, irrespective of age, and be counseled about the differences between screening and invasive diagnostic testing.

The introduction of DNA microarray technologies makes individual decisions about screening for each disorder impracticable and attempt at differentiating screening (i.e., interventions used to detect any anomaly or disorder in a population) and diagnostic testing (i.e. detection of a specific disorder in an individual patient) ineffectual. Massive amount of information of unknown importance will be generated, making information disclosure unrealistic, if not harmful. While genetic screening of adults allows time to rescreen to confirm findings and to interpret or ignore screening results, in prenatal care it might allow only weeks or even days for a critical decision on the viability of a pregnancy.

All screening methods produce both false positive and false negative results as above noted.[5] Furthermore, anomalies that would have remained hidden during a lifetime "as non-activated tendencies in the absence of environmental challenges, and thus could have been ignored,"[3] are now exposed, and examined. The search may be so extensive that no fetuses may be found to be "worthy of life." But even with a 100%accuracy this would not help because there is no such a thing as "perfect" genome since all humans are programmed for death. Such quest for a "healthy" fetus, and therefore a healthy baby may result in having none. The more detailed the search for defects, the less likely it is to produce information that translates into useful knowledge about the health of a fetus, and thus the future health of the child. There are anomalies that should not be revealed and findings that are to be left silent for the benefit of the pregnant patient and her future child.

These considerations led me to conclude in 2003 that "unless physicians take a firm position against the use of these new genomic technologies in the contested terrain of prenatal screening they will probably have to surrender to parental requests for screening and disclosure either because they incorrectly assume that consumer choice is equivalent to autonomy or because of unjustified concern over being sued for wrongful birth, (i.e., not having disclosed enough information to make an informed choice about whether to continue a pregnancy)."[4] This was, in essence, if not completely, the position adopted by Dr. Nisand, my colleague in Monaco, and against which I had argued, though in a different context. I came to realize that it was less about non-disclosure of genetic information than the manner in which non-disclosure was achieved that fueled my arguments. Physicians should not have the authority to decide unilaterally what and whether to disclose based on what they think is a "minor" or a "serious" fetal condition. This decision belongs to the patient informed by her physician. Judging a condition as minor or serious is highly subjective, i.e., it rests on the subject, or the person who makes a judgment; that which is minor to one person may be serious to another. The difficulty is to give these concepts an objective (i.e. scientific) content.

3. Fetal DNA sequencing

The completion of the human genome project, a decade ago, failed to bring about the therapeutic breakthroughs it promised. Except for a small number of genetic conditions, the predictive power of gene sequencing as been low and detailed catalog of gene expressions has been so far of little interest. Misha Angrist, (a pioneer in *Personal Genome Project* , who had his genome sequenced) noted: "Time and again, the paucity of genomic information was striking: I would find mutations in genes that coded for proteins but the proteins' ascribed functions would be so general and/or tentative as to be meaningless. In some cases, the proteins didn't even have names, let alone functions assigned to them."[5]

Regardless of paucity of success in assigning functions to proteins coded genes , research has intensified on successfully extracting cell free fetal DNA from maternal plasma samples in early gestation. Extracting cell free fetal DNA is difficult because these cells constitute less than 10% of total DNA in maternal plasma, and intact fetal cells are even less. The hope is that once fetal DNA can be easily (i.e. noninvasively), dependably and inexpensively obtained from maternal blood, it may be sequenced and would provide the genetic blueprint of a fetus, with actual and predictive power to reveal all that which may affect the health of the future child. George Annas has used the metaphor of "future diary" to illustrate it.

A close analogy to fetal DNA sequencing would be the "whole body scan," or the computerized tomography (CT) body screen, also called computerized axial tomography (CAT) screening. This CT Body screen has been marketed as a preventive or proactive health measures for asymptomatic ("healthy") individuals, to assist in detecting that which could potentially be harmful medical conditions. Theoretically, the whole body (CT) scan would permit a transparent view of the entire body and help detect harmful and deadly conditions in early stages, and therefore save lives. However, in practice, the risks outweigh the benefits. For example, risks may include a low rate of finding meaningful markers for actual diseases; confounding results because of "incidentolomas" or pseudo anomalies, i.e. anomalies that are often not related to any disease and which may be benign[6,7]; high costs of the procedure itself and the relatively high level of radiation exposure associated with it which may cause cancer later in life. No data have been presented to the FDA to demonstrate that the whole body CT scan is effective for screening or testing individuals without symptoms. FDA has not approved CT screen for whole body screening use. Nonetheless, physicians may decide that a asymptomatic patient may benefit from CT screening ("off-label" use of the medical device).

A similar scenario may unfold with regard to fetal DNA sequencing. This may create problems analogous to, but much more damaging than other methods of screenings, including DNA microarrays. Fetal DNA screens would combine questions similar to routine screening methods, but the complexity of the results will add new elements that make disclosure of fetal information and subsequent parental decision about the pregnancy much more complicated. Users of these screens may either (incorrectly) think that there is nothing more important to know about their fetuses than their genomes if it is for health preservation and avoidance of diseases or may (unjustifiably) oversimplify gene expression and the predictive power of DNA sequencing.

Deploying the whole fetal genome in prenatal practice is controversial and difficult to interpret.[8] It is controversial because it could be damaging to the future child since it does constitute the child's permanent medical record and may be used to discriminate against the child, once born. It may be misleading and falsely reassuring because of false positive and false negative findings. Moreover, patients are notoriously ignorant about genetics, and nonetheless, may request direct access to the fetus' genomic data, just as they may have direct access to their own genome. And geneticists, themselves are divided on what conditions should be considered serious, and have conflicted views on genomic findings, which limit their capability to reasonably inform and counsel their patients. Genomic data are difficult to interpret, and the time spent to sift out and interpret these data in way that could be meaningful to patients may be so enormous as to be impractical.

Direct- access to fetal genomic data may exacerbate these problems. Direct-to-Consumers genetic testing companies have used different strategies to minimize the difficulties inherent to the practice and help adults navigate their genetic screens. For example *23&me* and *Navigenics* have provided customers with inexpensive and easy to understand genetic information, including a basic understanding of the meaning of predisposition to specific disorders and ethnic ancestry, but have offered little scientific explanation. *Sciona* genetic firm has chosen to link genetic information to a customer's lifestyle, and *DNA Direct* supplies customers with access to qualified doctors to help interpret genetic test results. In all, profit rather than scientific knowledge has been the immediate driving force.

Genes operate through a series of instructions that may be spelled out, but cannot be fully predicted and explained. The deeper we delve into our genome, the more opaque it becomes. It may be possible to retrospectively determine what might have predisposed a person to actual disorders. But no model exists that may help to comprehensively predict how genes respond to challenges, interact with the environment and restructure themselves to ensure health and survival.[9] Genetic markers commonly associated with a specific disease say little about a future child's health or the seriousness of future diseases.

Nonetheless, prospective parents may request the whole genome sequencing of their fetuses, once it is feasible and affordable (or even if they must pay the extra cost) because they believe it will give them all the information they need about their babies' future health. Just as Bill Clinton, then president, believed it was a good idea to give parents at the birth of their newborn, a CD with the sequencing of the child's entire genome, we too believe that it is a good idea to give prospective parents a CD of fetal cell DNA sequencing that they may explore as the same time the fetus develops *in utero*. But, of course, there is a major difference between information that relates to a child having full legal and moral rights, including a right to privacy, and genomic information of a not- yet- born child having interests in life and health, but no right to be born. One may be seriously concerned at the prospect that prospective parents might select their future children by genetically auditioning them via fetal DNA sequencing, before permitting them to be born. And there are also questions about parents' rights to know and the child's right to privacy. What should physicians do to reasonably assist and counsel their pregnant patients? Should they respond positively to request by prospective parents and adopt a market-based genomic model or consumer choice? Should they remain neutral or should they take action to help ensure that fetal genomic information, if and when it is part of routine prenatal care, constitutes knowledge that is reasonably understandable and meaningful, and when put in a realistic context reflects the actual concerns of their pregnant patients? Of course there is always the option of not offering prospective parents whole genome screens of their fetuses because of the many confounding variants of uncertain or unknown clinical utility, validity, or significance. Results of these screens, if reported to the pregnant patient may caused a level of stress and anxiety that may put the pregnant patient and the entire pregnancy in jeopardy. However, this option strikes me as untenable, in a culture of "laissez faire" in assisted reproduction.

Other alternatives include offering routine genome screening of fetuses and let physicians decide what findings to disclose, based on professional standards developed by relevant medical practice standards committees – the *Professional Standards Model*, or letting the pregnant patient decide about whether to be screened and what information to have access to –the *Consumer Model.*

Professional Standards Model, gives physicians the authority to decide on disclosure of findings they believe may cause more harm than good, based on their medical judgment. This Model, in effect prioritizes harm- benefit assessment of genomic screens over the parental right to informed consent, and is based on the ethical concept of beneficence, Doing good. , i.e., a procedural mechanism that evaluates the overall benefit of the genetic intervention over harm. This Model substitutes the question of right to informed consent with a welfare question, i.e. what should be done to promote the best interest of patients. The first question is relevant to the pregnant patient; the second question is relevant to physicians who decide what should be done to protect the interest of patients. information and genetic findings are worth disclosing to the pregnant patients. It marginalizes (even displaces) the rights of prospective parents in favor of the welfare question and is mostly procedural rather than substantive. It conflates the concepts of autonomy (individual rights) and beneficence (doing good, maximizing benefits, minimizing harm).

The *Consumer Model* alternative leaves the decision about whether to be screened, and what information to have access to, to the pregnant patient. It is probably a model that is most consistent with American values since it favors individual right to autonomy and consumer choice, permits the pregnant woman to manage her pregnancy, decides whether or not to be screened, the amount of information she needs and whether and when to access this information. A genetic counselor is necessary before allowing access to genomic data and afterwards for interpreting these data. Because genomic information is inherently information overload, and the majority of genomic findings is not clinically useful or meaningful and readily applicable, patients will need to know in advance how deeply they want to delve into their fetuses' genome. This is an extremely difficult task, and virtually every geneticist - physician as well as expert commentator has insisted that anyone who wants to access genomic data must be accompanied by serious genetic counseling services. This makes sense.

One way to accomplish this task (which should be discussed, but currently strikes me as the most reasonable) would be to routinely offer fetal genomic screening and disclose information about the specific conditions which prospective parents themselves are most concerned about (e.g., Down syndrome, neural tube defect), including conditions that have caused pain, disability and suffering to previous children in the family. Other conditions may be disclosed such as those that have been qualified as "serious" by prospective parents, by a regulatory agency in terms of the disability, pain and suffering they cause (as in Britain) or by law because they are fatal at an early age, and incurable at the time of the screen (as in France). Exception to disclosure, could include, for example, conditions considered "serious" but predictably may develop in adulthood or late in life, such as breast cancer, Alzheimer's, Parkinson's etc… This is because, any documentation on these conditions may become part of an individual's medical record and could be used to stigmatize or even discriminate against the individual patient. This also raises the question of privacy protection right, or to put it another way, limits of parental rights to know.

Parents would have access to the remaining genomic data in the fetal genome (if they so desire), or could be provided with information attached, (e.g., via a website or flash drive), but only after they had undergone some education/counseling by a qualified genetic counselor. The counselor will assist patients after they have reviewed the genetic data themselves, and continue to assist them afterwards.

I favor this third model because it leaves the decision about whether to be screened, and what information to have access to, to the pregnant patient. This model recognizes the fundamental ethical principle of respect for persons, their rights to autonomy and self-determination within the doctor- patient relationship, but also taking into account the physician' s assessment of the patient's welfare and wellbeing. But this assessment does not trump the fundamental rights of the individual patient. This model is not the exact equivalent to consumer choice, nor is it paternalistic but should be viewed as a crucial part of informed consent.

Genome sequencing makes enormous amount of information available to pregnant patients who want it and are willing to responsibly undertake genetic education and counseling. Genomic data, put in context, can help pregnant patients make an informed choice about their pregnancies in accordance with their values and preferences.

There is a caveat, however. Because fetal genomic screens gives us access to information contained in the entire fetal genome, it may be less costly than using DNA chips or microarray technology. To then decide on the conditions we may want to screen for may be, therefore, counterproductive and counterintuitive. So, if choosing those specific conditions that should be disclosed is the recommendation, we may want to explore the reasons why, in the first place, we give legitimacy to genomic screens in prenatal care. These reasons may weaken as we discover that there are actually very few genetic conditions prospective parents may want to know about when they look at genetic screens of their fetuses, and these conditions do not require the sequencing of the entire genome; they may simply require good family history practice.

4. References

[1] Nisand MI. Procréation et nouvelles technologies: état des lieux. In AMADE-UNESCO, Proceedings of the International Symposium on Bioethics and the rights of the child, April 28-30, 2000; Monaco: 31-36.

[2] Nisand MI. Délai de l'IVG. Contre la réification du fœtus humain. http://www.femiweb.com/editorial/edito_core.htm (accessed 5/14/10)

[3] Canguilhem G. Te normal and the pathological. New York Zone Books, 1989

[4] Shuster E. Microarray genetic screening: a prenatal roadblock for life? The Lancet; 2007;369:526-529.
[5] Angrist M. Here is a human being. At the down of personal genomics. Harper Collings Publishers, 2011
[6] Kohane IS, Masys Dr et al. The incidentalome. A threat to genomic medicine. JAMA 2006;296:212-15
[7] Stone JH. Incidentalomas -clinical correlation and translational science required. N Engl J Med 2006;354:2748-49
[8] Berg JS, Khoury MJ, Evans JP. Deploying whole genome sequencing in clinical practice and public health: meeting the challenge one bin at a time. Genetics in medicine. 2011;13 (6):499-504
[9] Shuster E. Determinism and reductionism: a greater threat because of the human genome project. In Annas GJ, Elias S eds. Gene mapping: using law and ethics as guides. New York, USA: Oxford U Press, 1992:115-27